THE KAIZEN METHOD

TO LIVING A
HEALTHY LIFESTYLE

Lose Weight and Feel Great
with
Better Eating and Exercise Habits

BARBARA DEE

Printed in the United States of America.

Published by Suncoast Digital Press, Inc.

Sarasota, Florida

www.SuncoastDigitalPress.com

ISBN: 978-1-939237-29-3

Graphics by Zoe Radford

Contents

Contents

Foreword

By Harvey S. Mishner, MD

As the founder and CEO of the Kaizen Total Wellness Program, I am pleased to recommend this book to all of our patients, friends, and anyone looking for a practical and encouraging approach to improving their health. Rather than a "How To" or novel, this book will guide, motivate, and help you with a strategy you haven't seen applied to healthy habits before, yet it's been proven effective for decades.

Several years ago, I too got caught up in an unhealthy lifestyle consisting of too much work, eating too much sugar, and not exercising. Yes, it was always, "I'll start tomorrow." But one day tomorrow finally came. Utilizing the methods outlined in this book, I slowly changed my lifestyle. This meant healthier food choices, not diet or deprivation. It meant increased activities, not "exercise" (sounds too much like work).

After a few months, the pounds were coming off very quickly. Because I was so successful and it was so easy, we decided to offer this as the first stage of the Kaizen Total Wellness Program. We know that nutrition is very important, but too many people have their own misconceptions of what a diet should be. We still NEED sugars, fats and proteins, but the RIGHT sugars, fats and proteins.

Exercise will increase endorphins and serotonin, which will give you more energy and improve your mood. Exercise will also naturally increase natural growth hormones which are also a very effective anti-aging agent.

Consistent with my philosophy of health (smart choices, no gimmicks), Barbara explains in a very engaging style how anyone can benefit from using the kaizen approach.

Hopefully reading this book will help with a positive attitude about your health. Like they say in the golf world, visualize a bad shot and you have no chance of being successful; picture the ball going in the hole and the odds go up dramatically!

Good luck and please contact us if you have any further questions.

Dr. Mishner

Chapter One

Introduction:
Why the Kaizen Approach Always Works

Neal Peterson was radiant as he spoke to my daughter's graduating 6th grade class. He had recently completed the "Around Alone" race, a harrowing voyage considered to be the Mount Everest of sailing. He told his story, recreating his adventure with such intensity that it felt as if I were there with him, splashed mightily with freezing cold water, holes in my boots, and the mast and my body now dipping again and again under the churning water, under the huge swells.

How did he do it, sailing around icebergs, and eventually around Cape Horn, alone, in the boat he built himself?

"I sailed 195 days," he said, "one day at a time."

What do you truly want to accomplish—whether it will take a year or a lifetime—that you could start right now, knowing you are only committing to it for one day at a time?

"I sailed 27,000 miles one mile at a time."

—Neal Petersen, Captain of "No Barriers," after completing the Around Alone Race

Are you trying to get more exercise, lose weight, or quit smoking? If so, you're not alone—those are three of the most common New Year's Resolutions or goals people say they want to achieve.

Since we know that only a very small percentage of resolutions are actually accomplished, what has the biggest effect on a person's success or failure? Wouldn't it be extraordinary to know the one approach that contributes to success and improved health more than anything else?

If you are looking for a brand-new concept, a high-tech solution, or *Voo-Doo Diets for Dummies*, this book is not for you. This book takes the proven, ultra-successful management approach termed "kaizen" in Japan and shows how it works for any individual who embraces it with the intention of developing a healthy lifestyle and enjoying its many rewards.

The Sino-Japanese word "kaizen" simply means "good change" and refers to any improvement, large or small. In restoration efforts after WWII, it became common practice in Japan to label their emerging philosophy of productivity improvement "kaizen" and the method was famously and successfully adopted by Toyota.

The culture of continual, aligned small improvements and standardization yields large results and compounds productivity improvement. This differs from the "command and control" improvement programs of the mid-twentieth century.

Most of us are all too familiar with the shortcomings of the "command and control" method when it comes to changing eating habits, starting an exercise regimen, or even trying to count carbs, points, or calories. Even if discipline is maintained for a few short-term results, most often the results are not sustained.

So, with previous tries, you haven't achieved and maintained your desired level of health and fitness—but it is important to note that there are certainly other goals in life which you have achieved. How did you get so good at what you're really good at? It did not happen overnight. It did not happen without your intention and persistence. You mastered certain skills and succeeded with your learning goals through a series of steps, over time.

Healthy lifestyles are built out of small changes that become new patterns and habits.

We are creatures of habit, and when it comes to our health, that is good news. Brain researchers have discovered that when we consciously develop new habits, we create new brain cells and synapses. This means that our new *chosen* patterns of thinking and newly *chosen* habits become a part of us.

The kaizen method works in complete and harmonious alignment with the way our brain works. Small and continuous improvements are at the heart of small or big change, and when this is the path of change, it has been found that momentum is increased.

Imagine if you needed to change course while steering a large boat. If you slowed down enough to make a sharp turn, you would lose all momentum. Then you have to expend a lot of energy to overcome inertia and get back to making any forward progress. But if instead you made a *small* course correction, you would proceed in the new direction more gradually, but without losing momentum.

When it comes to making lifestyle changes, momentum is affected by things like motivation, optimism and the psychological will to change. One of the biggest drags on our momentum is fear. In her book *This Year I Will...*, M.J. Ryan writes, "Whenever we initiate change, even a positive one, we activate fear in our emotional brain. If the fear is big enough, the fight-or-flight response will go off and we'll run from what we are trying to do."

Our own mind can work against us! We say we want to develop healthier habits that would be good for us, and yet we are often guilty of self-sabotage.

Ryan notes that "*Small* steps don't set off fight-or-flight, but rather keep us in the thinking brain..." This is how we keep fear from taking over. Ah yes, Bob Wiley (played hilariously by Bill Murray) practiced this in the 1991 movie, *What About Bob?* As instructed by his psychiatrist, Bob verbally coached himself to take "...Baby steps get on the bus, baby steps down the aisle, baby steps..." In this manner he conquered his many fears and made slow and steady progress towards better mental health.

Ryan's advice echoes the kaizen approach of making small, steady improvements. As she explains, you want to stretch yourself out of your comfort zone, but not so far out that you experience stress, fear, or overwhelm.

Can you commit to that? Identifying small steps and then taking them? In the following six short chapters, you will learn how to name and take your next small step, and the next, as you develop healthier habits and embrace a healthy lifestyle. You will learn how to be consistent with your steps forward, and what to do when you find you've taken a step backward.

You've been saying you *want* to be healthier. Unfortunately, no matter how many times you say that, no matter how many people you say that to, and no matter how much you really mean it, it makes no difference.

For you to have any sustainable success, you need to shift from "I want to" to "I will."

> As your first baby step, start saying, "I will...."
>
> "I will go for a walk before I get ready for work."
>
> "I will choose the grilled salmon instead of the fettuccini tonight."
>
> "I will buy new running shoes that I love by the end of this weekend."
>
> "Just for today, I will set out eight bottles of water and drink them all."

Notice that these promises are all achievable and have a specific time attached. Your first assignment is to get a notebook and begin writing down your "I will" baby steps. See Appendix A for tips on setting up your healthy lifestyle notebook, forms you can use, and examples.

My Total Wellness *Journal*

The Kaizen Method to a Healthy Lifestyle   *Archer* Inspired Learning

Your notebook is your personal helper.

Name your notebook/journal in a way that draws you to it. Design it in a simple way that inspires you. It's just for you and only needs to make sense and be helpful to you, personally.

You'll be using this notebook for many different assignments as you progress through this book, all with the same purpose—to increase your awareness of your healthy lifestyle progress, which begins the moment you commit.

"To commit when I feel inspired, capable and grand is one thing... I will also commit on days when I feel dull, blue and insignificant."

—Eric Maisel, *Affirmations for Artists*

Chapter One Key Point: The kaizen approach works because you are making small, continuous changes. Your mind feels stretched, but not overwhelmed.

Chapter One Assignment: Consult Appendix A for tips on setting up your Healthy Lifestyle notebook. Write about your desire to lead a healthy lifestyle, as well as the challenges and excuses that have thwarted your efforts in the past. Make a fresh commitment, starting now.

For example, you may have a goal to lose a certain number of pounds. Research shows that simply writing down everything you eat and drink each day makes a huge difference to weight loss. Is that a step you are ready to take? What else might be useful to track? Using your notebook, no matter what format you find most convenient, will serve to increase your daily awareness and will accelerate your efforts while reducing effort and struggle. You can jump over to Appendix A now if you wish.

Chapter Two

Get Your Mind and Body to Work Together for Your Greater Good

Do you realize that you talk to yourself all day, every day? Thankfully not out loud, for the most part, right? Closely examine the conversations you are having in your head about your lifestyle habits, because they will drive your actions—or lack of actions.

Change the conversation—change your behavior. Yes, it's that simple!

There are volumes written about reframing your thoughts and changing your inner script which seems to direct your actions and your life. The power of thought is a topic that has inspired brilliant writing and teaching, and for good reason: You become what you believe yourself to be, and you believe what you hear, repeatedly.

We know labels create self-fulfilling prophecies. We ache for the child whose parent tells him every day he is clumsy or stupid, as we are afraid the child will accept it as fact, and never realize a more successful possibility. We come to believe what we hear and think. To alter your way of being, change what you believe by *choosing* the thoughts you want to think, again and again.

"Mental exercise," promoted widely as a healthy habit, has seduced millions of Sudoku and crossword puzzlers into justifying their sedentary behavior as a good way to ward off Alzheimer's. Being a Scrabble® addict myself, I don't mean to disparage the fascination and entertainment value of these activities. However, there is a more useful and life-altering way to fire up those sleepy brain synapses.

I call it "intentional optimism." This is the practice of noticing and constructing the thoughts and sentences in your mind. Strengthening this mental muscle is how we imagine better realities in the future, and motivate ourselves to pursue those desirable future outcomes.

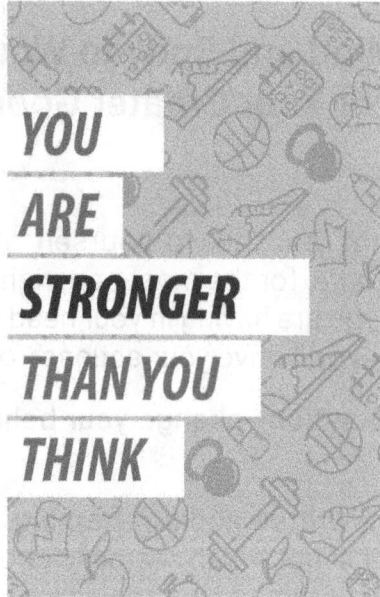

YOU ARE STRONGER THAN YOU THINK

Intentional optimism also has clear benefits in the present. Researchers studying heart disease patients found that optimistic patients were more likely than non-optimistic patients to take vitamins, eat low-fat diets, and to exercise, thereby reducing their overall coronary risk. A similar study of cancer patients revealed that pessimistic patients under the age of 60 were more likely to die within eight months than optimistic patients of the same initial health, status and age.

Some call it the power of positive thinking. Call it anything you want, just know that practicing this will help you develop and permanently adopt healthy lifestyle habits. With a healthy mindset, you will have more energy, more enthusiasm for life, lower health care bills, and a higher quality of life as you age.

CASE STUDY: A Kaizen Total Wellness patient, Thomas, had metabolic syndrome. That is, he had multiple health issues and was significantly overweight, had high cholesterol, and was on the dangerous edge of diabetes.

He came to the realization that he had enjoyed a lifelong romance with Italian food, and that he had been equating "healthy eating" with giving all of that up. With his old mindset, a good diet meant deprivation, boredom, and depression.

By focusing on changing his mindset first, Thomas succeeded in all of his health goals. In only six months, his lab results indicated he would not have to get prescription medications for cholesterol or diabetes, after all. He said that his weight loss had been "effortless." His secret? Thomas said, "Picnics."

Picnics? Thomas explained that he found a way to keep all the romance and enjoyment of cooking and eating delicious foods. By being intentional and creative, he used the festive and fun idea of a picnic to satisfy his emotional need for meal enjoyment. He planned, cooked and packed his favorite healthy foods, in the right quantities, into his picnic basket. Whether with friends or alone, he was completely prepared with a healthy meal, ready when it was time to eat. "Mangia! Mangia!"

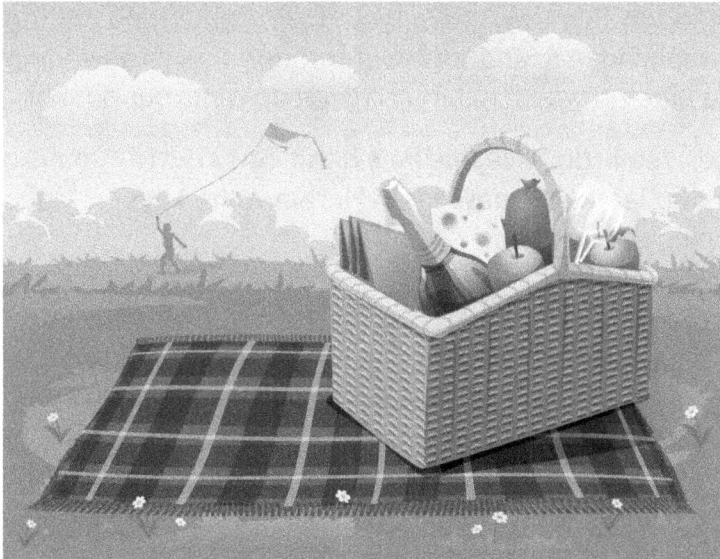

Starting with a healthy mindset is all-important when you want to effect positive change. Once you commit to the idea that it is not too late to learn something new, that an old dog can actually learn a new trick, you are on your way to better eating and exercise habits to help you feel great. To develop any new habit, there are only three things to put in place and 'Voila!' You can have any new habit you've been wanting to have.

Only three? Most of us can work with that, so I'll start with a short story illustrating the way these three keys work. When and I first moved to Sarasota several years ago, I stayed in my friend's guest house for a few weeks until I found our own place. It's a little house right by the side of her home. Her dear husband, so tolerant, came over to show me how to operate the TV, where to park, and when and how to take out the trash. The lesson on trash took an hour—this man has a <u>system</u>!

There are, not two, not three, but five different bins for garbage, each one a different color.

Being a grateful guest, I tried to pay close attention and I tried at all times to follow the rules, to remember to separate the waste, paper, glass, aluminum, plastic, plastic bags and donation items properly. I tried, and I succeeded, in developing the habit of recycling.

Compelled to this day, years later, I will fish a tuna can right out of the trash, rinse it, and walk out through the garage and plunk it into the blue recycle bin. I might even do it at *your* house!

You see, I really do have this new habit, one I did NOT have before. An old dog learned a new trick! Here are the keys to **S**uccess in developing a new habit:

1. Be clear on exactly what to do. I was **T**rained. I knew what I needed to do.

2. I was **A**ccountable. I knew my friend's husband came along behind me and corrected any category errors. I watched in horror one time as I saw him retrieve a Styrofoam cup I had stupidly put in with newspapers! I was lucky he didn't kick me out of the guest house.

3. I had built-in Rewards. I got to stay. I also had the satisfaction of doing the task right, and on time, each week. I could even tell I was getting better at it as time went on. And especially when I saw the big trucks come and take everything away, I felt like a part of a worthwhile effort. I was saving the Earth!

Let's see... **S**uccess: **T**raining—**A**ccountability—**R**ewards

I became a **STAR**!

You can be a **STAR** too!

Think of one habit you would really like to have in place, something that the consistent practice of would mean a higher quality of life for you, personally. A common one is to get more exercise.

Using the STAR keys, you know that to be **successful** in having a new habit of exercise, you would first need to understand exactly how to do it. I asked my personal trainer at Kaizen Total Wellness, what is an example of an exercise that is really important to do, but that people often do incorrectly? She quickly answered, "The Pec Fly."

Excuse me? She demonstrated. "The Pec Fly—you hold a light free weight in each hand, out to the sides, and slowly bring your hands together, then back out. Done properly, this is excellent for strengthening your pectoral muscles, helps your core, chest, arms, improves balance and stamina."

I asked, "What happens if you do it wrong?"

"Performed improperly, people extend too far back and put all the strain on their shoulders which could damage their joints and even tear their rotator cuff, which requires surgery to fix."

Okay, yes. I see that **training** is very important! Plus, don't we always feel more <u>confident</u> when we start doing anything new if we've been shown or told how to do it?

Then, there's **accountability**. Are you more likely to complete your workout routine if you have an appointment with a personal trainer or if you are home alone? Are you more likely to go for a long walk if you've planned to meet a friend and walk together?

Lastly, we need to build in some **rewards**. What trumps being lazy, sleeping in, skipping exercise? It is important to come up with *something*! New desired behavior needs to be reinforced with reward. One of my clients has a goal to put 10,000 steps on her pedometer every day for ten days, then she will buy herself the great new running/walking shoes she really wants. Or how about rewarding three weeks of consistently practicing your "new trick" with time at the beach, spa, or craft show?

Write in your calendar each time you will practice your new habit and at the end of three weeks 'X' out half a day for a treat you will love looking forward to.

Show yourself it's not too late to learn a new trick. It's the perfect time to start acting like the star of your own life. For **success**, just remember to make sure you are confident enough about what to do, or get any **training** you need. Then, design a way to be held **accountable** until the new habit becomes as automatic as brushing your teeth, and build in **rewards** for milestones along your way. Any new habit can be yours.

> **"Life isn't about finding yourself. Life is about creating yourself."**
>
> **—George Bernard Shaw**

Training starts with your mind. In your Healthy Lifestyle notebook (discussed in the previous chapter and explained in Appendix A), write a list of limiting thoughts and excuses that are running around in your mind waving a white flag of surrender whenever you try and push yourself a little. Notice these old conversations, the things you have been telling yourself about why you don't eat the right way or why you can't find time to exercise.

Writing these down and seeing these irrational discouragements in the light of day will help reveal what has been holding you back, and give you clues to what you want to adopt as your *new* way of thinking.

By managing the conversations you are having with yourself, your desired actions become much easier, almost **effortless**.

Recently, I was expecting my daughter to come home from college. All my thoughts gave rise to happy, excited feelings. When I heard her car outside, I sprang from the couch like a circus poodle and glided the 20 yards to greet her. Contrast this with someone sitting on the couch watching TV when a solicitor rings the doorbell. Their thoughts create feelings of annoyance and they might as well be in quicksand up to their knees. Sighing, standing up, and trudging to the door is so hard, so tiring, such a *pain*.

Have you ever had the thought "exercising is such a pain"? (If so, add this to your notebook as one of your limiting beliefs or old ideas.) What is the opposite thought? Perhaps "exercising is such a pleasure" or "exercising is the most fun part of the day." Did you just hear a scoff in your head when you read that? (If so, write that down in your notebook as another counter-productive thought.)

It is time to reprogram any old thoughts that do not serve you. One cannot simply wipe the slate clean and begin with all new healthy thoughts. You must DISPLACE the old with the new. That is, gradually bring in more and more healthy thoughts, literally crowding out the old, disempowering ones. After all, they are toxic and must be flushed out!

If you attempt to practice your new healthy habits without working to replace toxic thoughts with healthy ones, you're relying on willpower. Meaning, you *will* yourself to ignore the mind and "just do it." This can work, for maybe a week, but it is energy-draining and not sustainable. By following the kaizen method and each step outlined in this book, you will find developing a healthier lifestyle much easier than you ever thought possible.

STOP SAYING
TOMORROW

You'll take a few minutes at the end of this chapter to start writing the new thoughts you will choose to hear and believe, which will help you have and enjoy a healthy lifestyle. It is critical to your success for you to speak to yourself more encouragingly. It is just as important to stop fueling the old mind machinery which doesn't serve you. Notice those thoughts, record them if helpful, then say, "Thank you for sharing" and switch your full attention to the empowering thoughts instead.

Here are some examples, typically called "affirmations" because they affirm your commitment to intentional optimism. You may use these if you wish, and I also suggest you write your own.

Affirmations for Healthy People

- My mind and body work together for my greater good.
- Practicing my healthy habits bolsters my enthusiasm for life.
- I say "Yes!" to healthy activities—vitality is a function of participation.
- Moving my body releases stress.
- Being mindful today means more enjoyment today.
- I feel the rush of feel-good hormones as soon as I begin exercising.

- My life is becoming more disciplined, which is so freeing.
- I put in my mouth only what helps my body systems work well, including plenty of water.
- Gratitude and worry cannot coexist—I choose gratitude.
- Who is responsible for my health? I am.
- As I relax and clear my mind, intending healthy thoughts, I feel peaceful.
- I imagine my heart, tirelessly pumping life through my body. Thank you, heart.
- I imagine my lungs, expanding with my deep breath, and then exhaling any tension my body was holding. Thank you, lungs.
- I am flexible. If one plan for a meal or exercise doesn't work out, I easily find another good one.
- I persevere. If I skipped a healthy habit, I put that behind me and take the next right action.
- I choose to stay in balance. Healthy habits work in harmony with all my priorities.
- I am committed to progress, not perfection.
- I consciously design my home to support my healthy lifestyle.
- Leading a healthy life is very important to me. I will do my best.
- Every day I have time to play.
- The smallest step in the right direction builds my confidence.
- I am training my mind to choose healthy thoughts and to direct my body in healthy behaviors.
- I am a gentle reminder to myself, full of compassion.
- I plan ahead so my self-care is easier.
- There are plenty of people and resources to help. I can find support whenever I need it.
- I act as if I am a health-conscious person.
- I love my journey towards total wellness.
- One day at a time, I feel healthier and more alive.

Feel free to copy any of these into your healthy lifestyle notebook, giving yourself permission to change the wording and also create new ones. You can find additional examples online if you search for "health affirmations." Louise Hay has written dozens of books and articles on healing as it relates to the power of positive thought. Also remember the destructive power of negative thought which we can slip into when we start judging our less-than-perfect behaviors and become too self-critical. Better to shift from being *critical* to being *curious*. Catch yourself: *Hmm...I wonder where that thought came from. Kind of sounds like my overly-critical mother. Or, isn't this curious... I don't know how long I have been standing here in front of the refrigerator with the door open, staring inside.*

One of the best ways to instill affirming thoughts of choice is to read them out loud to yourself. Seeing and hearing them helps your mind remember them. That will help them take hold and edge out the automatic, reactive, toxic thoughts. Why not store your list of new thoughts right on your tablet, smartphone, or other handy device—it's a great way to help keep your empowering voice present. You need a "reset button" when the old thoughts take over. You have some brainwashing to undergo, but keep in mind the result is a cleaner bill of health!

Chapter Two Key Point: The self-talk and automatic thoughts you listened to in the past got you where you did *not* want to be, just like listening to new, health-minded encouragements will get you where you want to go. For success in developing a new habit, remember the acronym **STAR**. **Success** comes from having the proper **training**, being held **accountable**, and building in **rewards**.

Chapter Two Assignment: Write about your confidence level for a new healthy habit you would like to have. Is there some training (such as from a nutritionist or personal trainer) which could help you feel more confident and motivated? Do you have any structure of accountability such as a Wellness Coach or exercise buddy?

Begin a list of rewards you can treat yourself to which are consistent with your new healthy lifestyle—not like eating a box of chocolates! In your notebook write the title: My Affirmations. Start writing short, encouraging sentences that you desire to be true, even if you don't feel they are true at the moment. For example, it's fine to write "I put myself to bed every night before 11:00 p.m." if that is a habit you wish to establish, even if you have seldom practiced it in the past. Refer to the affirmations in this chapter for ideas and write your first five positive affirmations.

Chapter Three

Script Rewriting:
A Different Result Only Comes from Doing Something Differently

"If we do not change our direction, we are likely to end up where we are headed."

—Chinese Proverb

As humans we all face challenges and turns of events we cannot predict. With the kaizen approach, we'll be ready for unexpected bumps in the road to wellness. Let's peek into people's lives and see some of these strategies in use.

Becky gets benched.

Becky donned her workout clothes and new tennies and headed toward the gym in her apartment complex. A familiar little furry ball ran up to her ankles, dancing around. Holding the leash was Lilia, Becky's 88-year old neighbor, lonely for a conversation as usual. Lilia looked especially fragile that day and Becky motioned toward the nearby bench under an oak. They sat down for a chat and Becky never made it to the gym.

We start out with the best of intentions, but get sidetracked all too easily when it comes to practicing healthy habits like regular exercise and clean eating. It happens to everyone, can be discouraging and depressing, and can derail the self-care our bodies require. There is so much at stake—our very quality of life—that it is worth learning and practicing new, health-conscious scripts to get us back on track.

Let's ask Becky to script the end of this episode in a way that fulfills her desire to get moving. This also demonstrates how to use intentional optimism to master and maintain healthy habits. Becky's new story ending:

Becky found herself sitting on a sidewalk bench instead of a gym bench. The little dog, Bella, danced around her feet. She remembered her much-practiced affirmation: "Living a healthy lifestyle is very important to me. I will do my best." She said to Lilia, "Bella has so much energy. How about if you sit here in the shade while I take her for a little jog around the apartment complex?" Lilia gratefully agreed and Becky set off for her jog. When she returned 25 minutes later, Lilia thanked her for letting Bella get some much-needed exercise. Becky smiled and walked with a bounce back to her apartment.

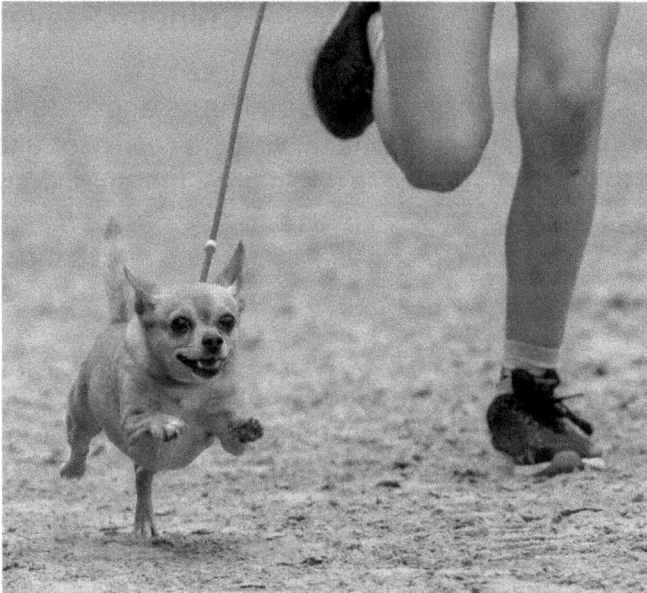

Becky's encouraging self-talk came into her mind effortlessly because she had trained herself with affirmations. Becky's story also reminds us to keep looking for opportunities to fit in healthy habits rather than letting a bump in the road justify the *reasonable* response to give up the journey. The opposite of being reasonable is not being unreasonable—it's being *intentional.*

Harrison's hunger hangs him up.

Harrison worked late, but still stopped at the grocery store as planned on his way home. He'd just returned from a business trip and had to stock up on just about everything.

Starting in the produce section, he selected a large variety of organic fruits and vegetables, and then progressed to the meat counter. After awhile, he chose the lean, skinless chicken breasts. By this time, he was noticing a piercing headache coming on, the kind he always got if he hadn't eaten for too long. He put his buggy into high gear and grabbed his whole grain bread, almond butter, low-sodium soy sauce and organic milk. Harrison prided himself on being a scrupulous label reader and only buying healthy foods.

Standing in the check-out line, he glanced at his watch, having a little trouble focusing through his headache strain. 9:15 p.m.! He had been in the store over 40 minutes. He hurried out to his car, feeling almost too weak to carry his three bags of groceries. As he pulled out of the parking lot onto the parkway, he saw the golden arches, that most familiar brand icon in the world. Realizing it would be almost two hours until he got home and finished preparing his food, he swerved into the right-turn lane, coming dangerously close to side-swiping a car, and continued his turn into McDonald's. He had barely pulled away from the drive-through window when he tore open the box, gripped the burger and took a bite of what was to be his 960-calorie meal, complete with 53 grams of fat and 1,336 mg of sodium.

Does this situation sound familiar? Life happens and our best intentions are waylaid. That is why we must practice our kaizen method until it comes automatically.

Let's ask Harrison to script the end of his story using tools and practices from the kaizen approach.

When Harrison arrived at his apartment, he was feeling much better, and much worse. He was no longer weak with hunger, but he was angry with himself for getting so desperate that he ate food totally out of sync with his healthy eating style. Luckily, he remembered these affirmations:

1. *My healthy habits work in harmony with all my priorities.*
2. *Who is responsible for my health? I am.*
3. *I consciously design my home to support my healthy lifestyle.*
4. *I plan ahead so my self-care is easier.*
5. *I am committed to progress, not perfection.*

More importantly, he thought of a very important tool I call the "Magic Question": What's my one next right action? And he immediately thought of some achievable steps to move him towards his healthy lifestyle goal. After putting away his groceries, he sat down at the kitchen table and started writing two lists: 1. Healthy Staples and 2. Snacks To Go.

The next day on his way home from work, he stopped to buy everything he wanted to never run out of (healthy staples). He included five frozen entrees which, after reading the nutrition labels, he deemed suitable and convenient alternatives to drive-through food when he needed a quick dinner. He also stocked up on his favorite low-sugar, high-protein snack bars, and cocoa-roasted almonds. He would put these in his travel briefcase as well as in his desk drawer at work. He knew he was infinitely more likely to eat when he first felt his energy getting low if he had healthy choices handy.

Like Harrison, you can set yourself and your environment up for success. You know you are busy and naturally have other priorities besides self-care, no matter how committed you are to living a healthy lifestyle. Make it as easy as possible to follow your healthy eating and exercise plans by creating an environment which really helps you.

How much thought have you given to setting up your environment to be healthy-habit friendly? Do you have water and healthy snacks handy whether you are traveling, playing golf, watching a ball game or driving in your car? Is there a TV by your home treadmill where you can watch your favorite show while getting in 30 minutes of great exercise?

Do you have a "purpose-driven" kitchen (see Appendix B for how to create one), full of only good choices and organized around delicious healthy recipes?

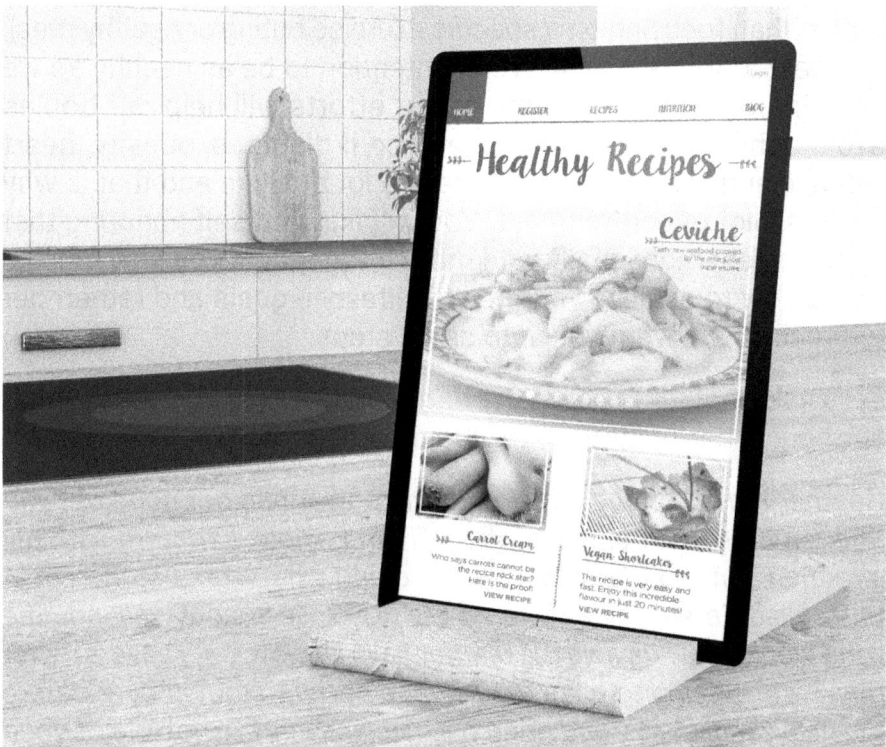

There are so many things that we have *no* control over which can throw us off track—be sure and pay attention to everything you *do* have control over. By planning ahead, you will have a much easier time mastering a healthy lifestyle.

Heather weathers the storm.

Heather set her alarm and placed her walking shoes next to her bed. She wanted to be ready to head out when her buddy Karen stopped by for their Saturday morning walk. In a still-dark room, Heather opened her eyes, awakened not by her alarm, but by a loud clap of thunder. Hurricane Maggie must be near, she thought, and sighed as she realized there would be no walk with Karen.

Even when we are willing and able, we can suddenly be thrown off our healthy habit track by life's circumstances, and should not expect otherwise. We can learn what to do when that happens, using simple tools and the kaizen approach.

Rather than focusing on a specific exercise outing or healthy meal, it is best to focus on our overall intention to be as healthy as we can, and on how the results of our efforts will help our bodies avoid debilitating diseases like Type II diabetes, obesity, heart disease and hypertension. There is a lot at stake and that is why it takes a lot of commitment. You will find yourself honoring that commitment more easily, and more frequently, if you stay flexible about how to achieve your healthy lifestyle goals and remember to break down every goal into small steps.

Let's ask Heather to script the end of her story in such a way that she honors her intention to maintain her new chosen healthy habits.

Heather turned on the lamp, glad the power had not gone out yet. She remembered her affirmation: "I am flexible: I am firm with my intention, but flexible with my plan, doing what works at the time." She called Karen who answered with, "No, we are not walking—the wind would blow us away!" Heather said, "I know, but I have a better plan—we're going to have a hurricane party! Come on over before the heavy rain starts, and bring candles and ice. I've got lots of good food and snacks. Bring your work-out clothes and when the power goes out we'll use the boom box and dance to CDs." Karen loved the idea of having fun with her friend, not riding out the hurricane alone, and taking advantage of "found" time to do healthy activities.

With one quick phone call, Heather took a key next action which set her up for success.

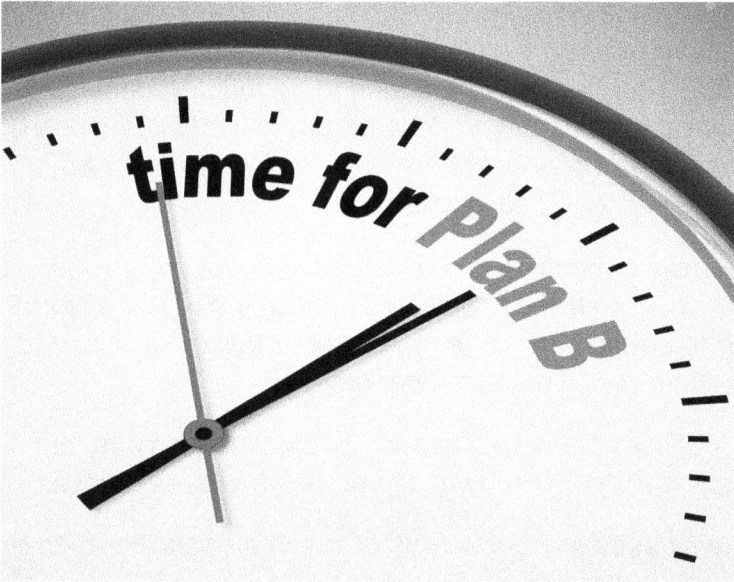

Why was Heather able to come up with such a great "Plan B" so quickly? First, she was focused on her intention of getting results versus being stuck on a certain plan of how to get the results. Secondly, she has a buddy with the same intention and healthy mindset. There is absolutely no use wasting energy trying to get someone to play healthy when they are not in the same game as you. She rightly guessed Karen would go along with the alternate plan which would provide the healthy activity they both wanted. Heather finds it empowering to remember she is not alone.

Terrie talks tough.

Saturday, after diligently walking/jogging 40 minutes every morning, six days a week for three months, Terrie had come in 1st place in her age group in the Manatee Park 5K Fun Run. She not only had the T-shirt, she had the toned legs and butt, and enough lung capacity to make it up the office stairs, rewards she noticed and appreciated.

Yet by Monday, the high from her victorious run had worn off, and the thought of getting ready for work was a total buzz kill. Her early alarm went off, set for her training routine. But instead of swinging her legs over the side of the bed and slipping her feet straight into her jogging shoes, she lay still, staring up at the ceiling. The conflicting thoughts in her head were too loud to permit drifting back to sleep. One voice said: Get up and do your run. The other whispered: Don't get up. You're too tired. There is no reason to keep training; you accomplished your goal on Saturday.

There was no more race on her calendar to look forward to, no event to train for, no goal she had shared publicly, no urgent and important reason to get up early. She rolled over, moved her pillow to shield the morning sun, and closed her eyes.

As a student of the kaizen approach to developing and maintaining a healthy lifestyle, Terrie wrote her new script as follows:

Terrie was suddenly conscious of warm air near her face and the purr of Stella, her cat.

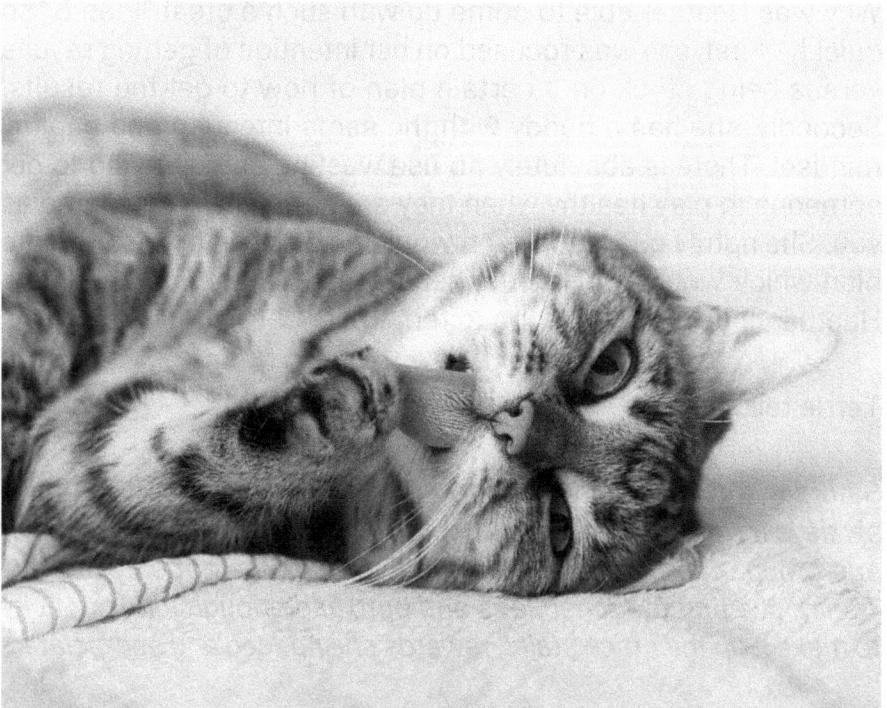

She was still in bed though the room was bright with sunlight, because she had decided not to do her morning run. Terrie wondered if she was going to have to sign up for another race in order to motivate herself to train. Then she remembered her goal—she was determined to lose 40 pounds by her 40th birthday, when she would throw a party called "Forty, Fit and Fabulous!"

It was 11 weeks away and she had 9 pounds to go. She pulled out her Healthy Lifestyle journal she kept by her bed, and reviewed the progress chart with the big smiley face she had added when she had gotten halfway to her goal. She read her 'Top Ten Reasons I Will Lose 40 Pounds' and the motivational quotes she had collected for inspiration. She focused on how much better she felt already with her 31 pounds gone. ("Gone forever!" she said in the mirror every morning.) She closed her eyes and took a deep breath and enjoyed her revitalized sense of purpose. She stepped in front of the mirror and said confidently, "You can do it." She put on her shoes, laced them up and ran her familiar route, noticing the new pink and green azalea buds.

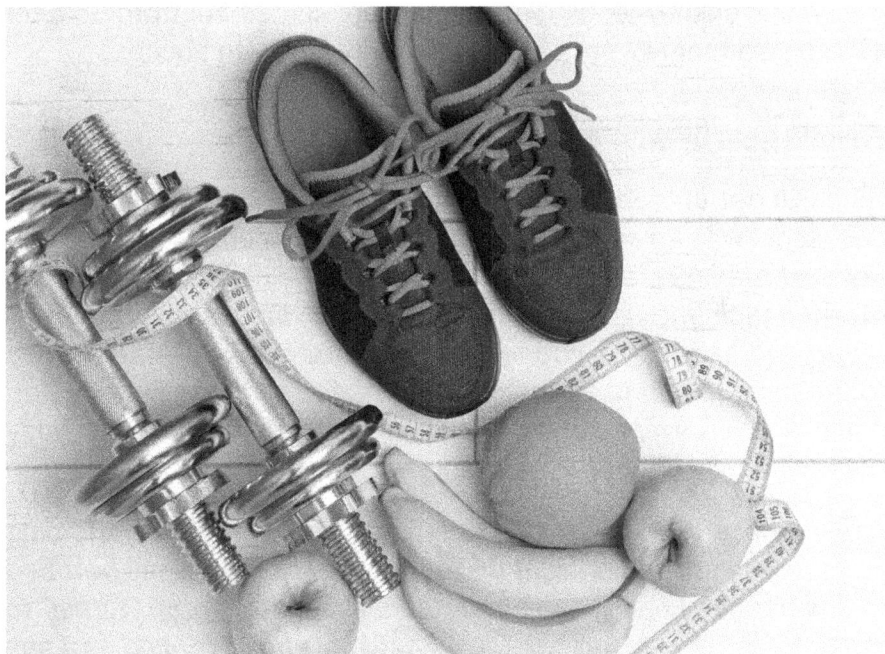

Terrie's story reminds us:

- **Set a goal that means a lot to you.** It can't be someone else's goal, not even your doctor's. It must be your personal goal, one that makes sense in terms of time and results, and one that you have a lot of reasons to accomplish. Remembering **why** you want to reach your health goals is the key to activating your motivation when you feel unmotivated. Imagine how you will look in that stretchy dress in six months. Think of what you will do with the extra $80 you won't need for medication every month when your doctor says you no longer have to take it. Picture yourself on a walking tour of London without getting tired or breathless.
- **Create milestones along the way.** A journey of a thousand miles begins with the first step. To take that step, you may need to have your sights set on the end of your street, where you will sit and rest and have a cool drink of water. Perfect. Find a small-step goal that your mind doesn't argue with. No matter how small it is, build your confidence by reaching and acknowledging each one step. Remember from Chapter Two that rewards along the way are key to success.

Frannie gets by with a little help from her friend.

When Janet invited Frannie to her first "Zumba" class, Frannie guessed it was an art or collage workshop, something like she and her best friend Janet had done before. To Frannie's delight, Zumba meant dancing to upbeat Latin music and watching the moves of Mario, the handsome young instructor. Frannie moved her body to the beat, laughing when Janet managed to catch her eye and smile. She left every class feeling invigorated and happy, her body unintentionally but nevertheless well-exercised.

Already looking forward to the next day's class, one Tuesday morning Frannie walked out her front door to mail a letter and was horrified to see her cat, Freeman, dead in the street. She never returned to Zumba class. It was too painful to imagine dancing around as if she were happily enjoying life...she wasn't.

How did the kaizen approach help Frannie? Her story continues...

Frannie called her friend Janet, tearfully relaying the tragic loss of her cat, and told her she would not be joining her at the Zumba class. Janet went over to Frannie's the next day after Zumba, bringing a bouquet of flowers and a sympathetic ear. The next Wednesday, Janet returned and asked Frannie to walk around the block while they talked. Frannie always felt better talking with her friend and readily agreed. This began a regular walk, which turned into a walk/ run, and one year later remains a weekly habit for the friends who have worked up to five miles every Wednesday.

Frannie's story reminds us:

- **Be gentle with yourself.** Just because you don't keep up a particular healthy habit doesn't mean you are doomed to weight gain and a heart attack. And it doesn't mean you are a lazy, weak person. It is simply that life is constantly changing, and when you surrender to that, you can remain in the flow and find yourself reaching your goal in a different way.
- **You are not alone.** Having a buddy is enormously helpful when developing new eating or exercise habits. In fact, to maintain those habits you may need lots of buddies. Be someone else's buddy and you'll see how much of an effective and mutually helpful tool this is. Remember from Chapter Two that accountability is one of the keys to developing a new habit.

Chapter Three Key Point: We have to take life as it comes, and we can use many tools to help us be healthy even when challenges arise.

Chapter Three Assignment: In your healthy lifestyle notebook, write a short account of a time when your healthy living routine was disrupted, like the situations above. Recall and write down how you reacted. If your response was less than ideal, write a new script of how you could have done it differently.

Chapter Four

Rounding Out Your Wheel of Wellness

Wellness is about more than diet and exercise. In fact, it would serve you to eliminate the word "diet" from your vocabulary. Diets do not work! Yes, you lose weight, but usually muscle and fluids, not fat. And about 95% of people who lose weight by dieting will regain it in 1-5 years.

Also, the deprivation of restrictive diets often leads to binge eating, another aspect of the unhealthy practice of "yo-yo" dieting where a person's weight goes up and down and the slowed-down metabolism and body systems are worse for the wear. Additionally, fad diets can be harmful, even fatal. They usually lack essential nutrients. For sure they teach you nothing about healthy eating, so when you inevitably go off the fad diet, the unhealthy eating patterns bring the weight right back and usually even more of it.

The best answer to healthy, sustainable weight loss is to learn about proper nutrition, meal frequency and food quantities, and begin your lifelong program of everyday healthy and pleasurable eating, along with regular exercise. And if the word "exercise" makes you frown, perhaps the idea of "moving your body" could make you smile.

Going back to our discussion in Chapter One about how our brains work, we know that often the words "diet" and "exercise" have come to connote such unpleasantness that they trigger fear and the instinct to flee. Even though at some level you want excellent healthy habits around food and fitness, we've all run away from perfectly good advice at times.

That's why this book is not about what to eat and how to work your body. This book is about being able to embrace good information, be motivated to practice it, and effortlessly continue to improve your lifestyle.

Picture a wellness continuum with extreme illness and disease at one end, and high-level, energetically optimal wellness at the other. With the kaizen method, you can see yourself making continuous, steady improvements along the continuum towards a higher and higher level of health.

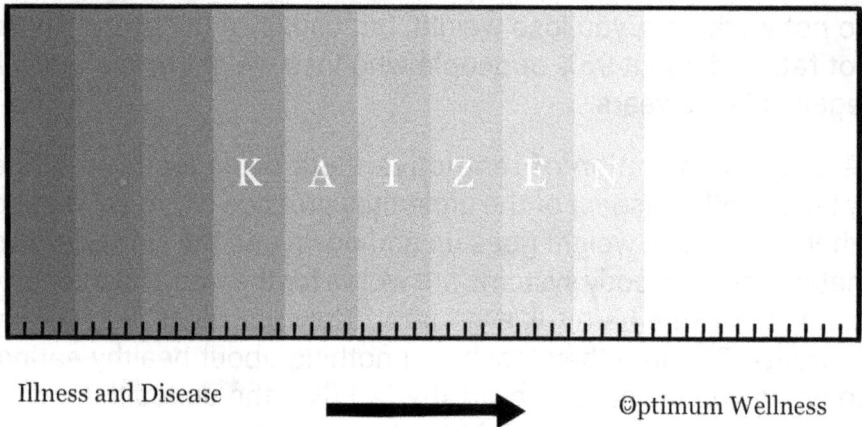

Illness and Disease   ⟶   ℗ptimum Wellness

There are many different domains in life which can be measured on a similar continuum, and you can gauge where you are in each of them. Wellness is multi-dimensional and each area, while it can be individually targeted for improvement, is part of the whole. Any gains or losses in one area will affect the whole.

The Wheel of Wellness (see Appendix C for an illustration) is an assessment tool that helps you measure your wellness in all areas of life. The wheel is divided into equal-sized pie slices with labels such as:

Health	Career	Money

Physical Environment Significant Other/Romance

Personal Development/Growth

Family	Fun & Recreation	Friends

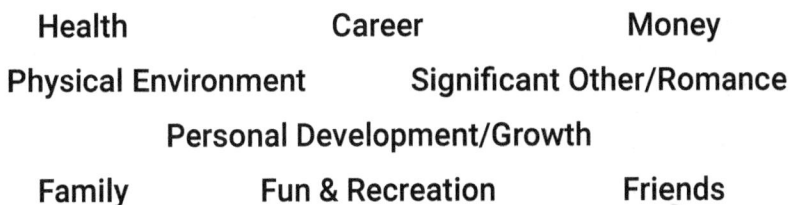

The different sections of the wheel represent holistic balance. When you measure your success in each area, you will notice that your scores are higher in some areas than others. You can see exactly which areas need attention in order to bring you towards total wellness.

The nine labels above are examples but you may use any label which means something to you, something that names a priority area or role you play. You may want to use fewer categories. See Appendix C and then create your own **Wheel of Wellness** in your notebook.

Draw your wheel with the number of equal-sized pie slices correlating to your list. Write the number '1' at the center of the wheel circle, and the number '5' on the outer edge of the wheel.

For each area, ask yourself how satisfied you are right now. Are you are devoting enough attention to this area? On a scale of 1-5 (1=LOW, 5=HIGH), notice your confidence and satisfaction, one area at a time, and draw a line across the slice at that level. You may end up with some long slices and some short slices. The wheel will take on its own shape, and unless you are a '5' in every area, you have been having quite a bumpy ride!

By shading in the pie slice up to your current level, you will literally see the gap between where you are and where you want to be. While you may not be sure exactly how to close the gap, you can commit that you will do your best. How can you round out your Wheel?

Ask yourself the Magic Question: **What's my one next right action**?

If the action seems too big, break it down. Don't let yourself get blocked by facing too big a leap. What's the baby step? Ideally you will stretch a bit to take this first step, but you can also look for a series of small, easy steps. Warren Buffet, the self-made billionaire, shared this: "I don't look to jump over 7-foot bars; I look around for 1-foot bars that I can step over."

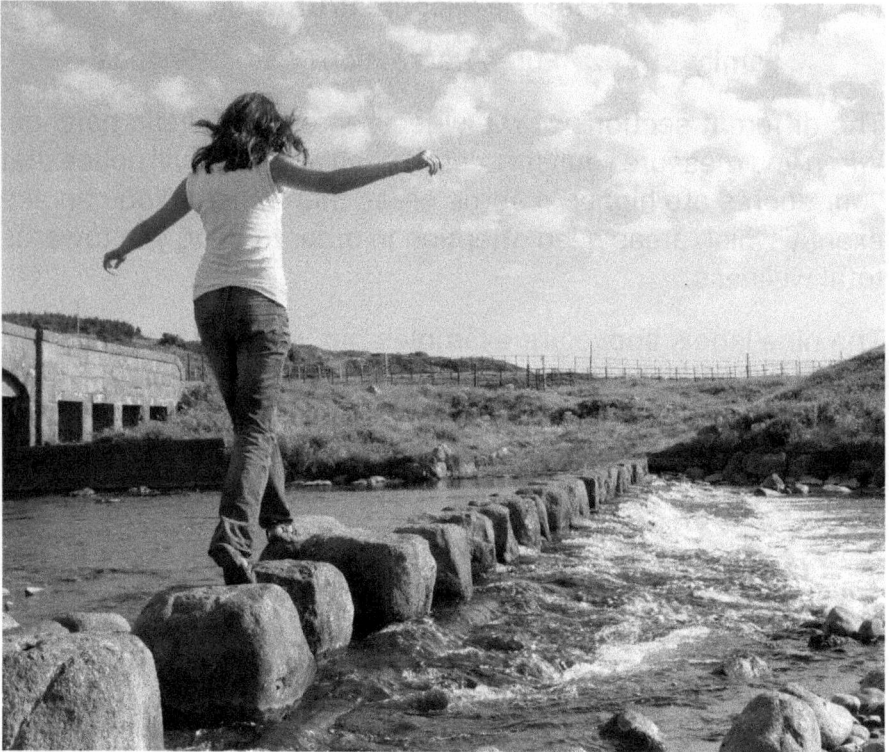

Here are **examples of small steps** in each of the example nine life areas:

Health & Well-Being

Buy a juicer. Set my tennis shoes and socks by my bed. Remove all the clothes hanging on my treadmill. Schedule a mammogram. Write down my body measurements in my notebook. Visit one yoga class.

Career

Print out my old resume to look at. Put a post-it on my computer reminding me to check *Craig's List*. Order the book *Take Yourself to the Top* by Laura Berman Fortgang. Sign up for the Real Estate course.

Money

Make an appointment to see my accountant. Set up a file folder to collect receipts I can turn in for reimbursement. Put all my credit cards in my sock drawer. Write an email to Nikki about the money she owes me. Post my extra china for sale on eBay.

Family

Send an e-card to Aunt Martha for her birthday tomorrow. Stop by the produce stand and get Molly's favorite sweet corn to make for her. Buy a frame for Andy's graduation photo. Send Josh a care package. Send Ave the fishing photos.

Friends

Write a thank you card and send to Teresa. Call Judy and set a tennis date. Call David and ask how Karen's surgery went. Return Dawn's paddle board. Create an e-vite with Denise's shower party info.

Significant Other/Romance

Check my frequent flyer miles and possible flights to Montreal. Ask Dick and Mary over for dinner. Plant the rose bush for Claire. Go to Victoria's Secret when I pick up my suit at the mall. Work on scrapbook ten minutes. Put love note in Terry's truck.

Personal Development/Growth

Clear bookcase of old books so I can choose and buy new ones. Write my "morning pages" tomorrow for five minutes. Check the ICF website and find three life coaches to interview. Find a Toastmasters club.

Fun & Recreation

Ask Maddie about going to Turtle Beach this Sunday. Purchase the pool basketball set Felton recommended. Look for my bowling bag in the garage. Call Debbie about dance music for the party. Book flight for Labor Day. Go see Deb at Comedy Club.

Physical Environment

Clean out the refrigerator. Stop by Salvation Army and empty my trunk. Spend five minutes clearing off my desk. Go to Staples and buy a new office chair. Order shades for the bedroom. Vacuum the car. Organize books by category.

If wellness is your desired destination, there is no better way to walk your path than to look at different domains of your life and apply the kaizen method of taking small steps. Feel free to use any of the above examples, change them to suit you, or write new ones. You can always change or rename the life areas. For example, if you're self-employed you may want to replace *Career* with *Business*.

Chapter Four Key Point: Forget "diet and exercise" and simply look at all areas of your life to see where you need to pay attention. Then ask yourself **what is the next one action to take**.

Chapter Four Assignment: Identify the areas of your life which, as a whole, encompass a balanced life as you see it. Look at the example in Appendix C and create your own Wheel of Wellness in your notebook. For each area, look honestly at where you are now and write down **one small step** towards where you want to be.

Chapter Five

Lighten Your Load to Gain Momentum Towards Wellness

Want more daily healthy energy? It does not come in a little can.

Power naps. A cup of coffee. A Snickers bar. There are all kinds of quick fixes we use when we've run out of energy but need to keep going. The success of the Energizer Bunny ad is surely because everyone longs to keep our own batteries charged, postponing the drain and staying up-and-at-it as long as possible—for the afternoon, or for our lifetime.

Energy is vitally important not only for your productivity and success in life, but for your health and happiness. Since we cannot plug ourselves into a power charger, and we know the caffeine will wear off, what's the best way to just feel like we have all the energy we need, to feel we are up to the task at hand?

Conventional wisdom tells us we can build stamina through exercise and cardiovascular improvement. True—yet feeling energized is not just a function of having a strong body. Just ask an athlete who has lost the ability to focus and consequently the ability to perform. Or think of a time when you felt emotionally or mentally drained during a challenging time in your life, or after a grueling test. Physical ability is only one ingredient of the recipe for having available energy.

The kaizen approach offers a deceptively simple yet very powerful practice for freeing up energy. The truth is that it's not only these big draining events in life we should think about, it's the little things we keep putting up with, stepping around and over. They pile up and weigh us down, draining our energy faster than we could possibly replenish it. Eliminating these tolerations will guarantee the recovery of that energy.

Examples of tolerations

I get a headache every afternoon. I have not talked with Beth in two years. My assistant calls in sick too much. I always forget to take my Vitamin D. My brother owes me money. My favorite pants are missing a button. The two prints I bought need framing. My husband dented my car and hasn't fixed it. My closet is crowded with clothes I don't wear. My cousin only calls me when he is drunk. My tennis racket has broken strings. My kitchen is full of junk food my wife buys.

Every little thing in your life matters; anything you are putting up with is taking a toll on your ability to function optimally. Even seemingly small things accumulate into a strong pull against your progress, like an anchor does for a boat, and cause you to feel just as stuck.

By becoming aware of these annoyances, these small or big things you are tolerating, you will see right away how they are having a cumulative effect on your quality of life. By spending just a little time noticing and cleaning up what you are tolerating, you will experience an immediate boost in your energy. (And you need this boost to empower your new healthy habits!) It's like you're lightening up the anchor and sailing forward with more and more speed.

Once you've identified and eliminated all your tolerations, you can pull up the anchor completely, catching the wind of wellness and sailing more easily through each day. I suggest you keep this picture in mind as you approach this assignment, as a gentle reminder of the importance to address each and every one of the tolerations that are weighing you down.

Other benefits of addressing tolerations

Handling a toleration causes us to focus on the *present*—it pulls us out of the past or future and has us be right in the moment, as a way of **practicing mindfulness**. Another personal benefit to this undertaking is that you will grow as a person. You will become more empathetic toward others, and more understanding of strengths and weaknesses, especially your own.

As a **more conscious person**, you will start to see what you *can* change, what you *cannot*, and what you need to accept. For example, with more compassion, you will find a way to *not* be drained by being around certain people, or, you will simply choose to *not* be around them.

Handling tolerations is good **Feng Shui**. Feng Shui is the practice of paying attention to energy: the flow of it, the lack of it, the harmonizing of it. Feng Shui teaches that when an area of your life is stagnant or troubling, it is beneficial to look for the cause and make adjustments, mainly in the way you have organized your home and yourself, to remedy life's annoyances and have a more vibrant life.

Handling tolerations helps you **simplify your life** and declutter your space, your calendar, and your mind. You will be clearing out the clutter of behavior patterns that have prevented you from living the life you really want. As you handle tolerations, you are moving away from procrastination and indecision, and you will enjoy more **clarity** and **inspiration**.

Once you start making your list of things you have been putting up with, you will uncover more and more, and it may seem a little overwhelming. It is very important that you freely add anything and everything you think of; don't get hung up on the next step of actually dealing with them. Just naming your tolerations frees up energy. Write it down even if you think you'll never be ready or able to handle it. As you keep identifying and addressing these things, after a short time you will definitely notice more natural energy. After a few weeks or months, you will see the light at the end of the tunnel and glimpse the possibility of a life free of tolerations, flowing with energy.

> **"Our tolerations are a mirror of what's going on inside us."**
>
> **– Thomas Leonard, Author, Coach**

Chapter Five Key Point: By noticing and eliminating things in all areas of life you've been tolerating, you will increase your energy, joy and health.

Chapter Five Assignment: In a separate section in your healthy lifestyle notebook, begin listing what you have been putting up with. It may be helpful to start with headings from each of your Wheel of Wellness domains from the previous chapter. As you review your notebook every day, look at this list and choose a toleration that seems easy to deal with. Decide what the first action step is towards eliminating that toleration. The item could be big such as "get a new job" or relatively small like "sew button on so I can wear my favorite pants." Tackle only the first step, not the entire item.

With the kaizen approach, you will address your list in tiny bites, making small, steady improvements in your life which will significantly increase your vitality.

Chapter Six

It's About Time

"There is so much time and so little to do!"

—Willie Wonka

Certainly one of the top excuses for neglecting healthy habits is not having enough time. And that's all it is, a dirty little excuse. Don't worry, I'm not going to tell you to just start making time for exercise or your other new healthy habits.

The truth is that you cannot make time, find time, manage time, lose time or save time. Some people say that good time management is about getting more done in less time. If you believe this, please stop. It doesn't serve you nor your commitment to living a healthy lifestyle. To best utilize our daily gift of time, we must **prioritize** what there is to do, and focus on completing the priorities.

This is why "to do" lists don't really work. Yes, we've asked you to make lists as part of this practice, and they do serve to get things out of your head and onto paper where you can see and act on them. But without prioritizing, how do you know if the next item on your list is going to be the most useful in helping you reach your goal of living a healthy lifestyle?

That's one reason for the Magic Question: **What's my one next right action**? To know what is "right" you must know your priorities, i.e., which action will further your highest priority commitments.

Credit is usually given to the late Stephen Covey (who was an extraordinary personal development expert) for a very powerful demonstration of prioritizing called "the big rocks exercise." Or you may have seen another time-management seminar leader use this memorable visual: He pulls out a large wide-mouthed jar and sets it on a table next to a small pile of fist-sized rocks. After filling the jar to the top with these rocks he asks, "Is the jar full?" Seeing that no more rocks would fit, the onlookers reply, "Yes!"

"Not so fast," he cautions. He then reaches beneath the table and pulls out a cup of pebbles from under the table. He pours them all into the jar, filling in the spaces between the rocks. Again he asks, "Is the jar full?" This time the audience replies, "Maybe not." The presenter produces a small bucket of sand and empties that into the jar, filling in the spaces between the rocks and gravel. "Is the jar full?" he asks. The audience, now fascinated, rightly guesses "No!" Finally, he grabs a pitcher of water off a side table and pours it in, filling the jar completely.

It is easy to imagine that if all the jar contents were on the table at the beginning, you might try pouring in the sand first, then a layer of pebbles and water. But then you'd probably only be able to fit one or two of the big rocks. So unless you do your most important activities **first** (the "big rocks"), it is unlikely you can fit them in later.

The point to remember is that by making a healthy activity such as exercise your "big rock" and fitting it into your day, the extra energy and vitality will allow you to fit more into your life. Instead of resenting the exercise as an interruption of your day, see it as the key priority that will help you do everything else.

Although there are some advantages, you don't have to do your healthy habits first thing in the morning; it's about consistently putting them in your daily planner until they become as automatic as brushing your teeth. Mark them down in your calendar as important appointments you keep with yourself. Besides being accountable by keeping these appointments, you will start to find many ways to include healthy habits in your normal routine without taking any extra time at all.

Expanding your activity literally does not have to "take" any time at all. Learn about the multitude of stretches and exercises you can do while you are "busy" on the phone, watching TV, or sitting at your desk. Here are a few you should become familiar with and give a try—they'll help get your blood moving, prevent stiffness and injury, burn calories, re-energize you, and build up balance and strength: arm circles, triceps dips, chair squats, calf raises, leg lifts, standing on one foot, finger stretches, neck rolls, and chest stretch. And for women, the Mayo Clinic recommends Kegels.

Start a list in your notebook of ideas like using a headset so you can stretch, walk and move around whenever you are talking on the phone; or bringing healthy snacks to work instead of frequenting the vending machine. With a kaizen mindset and the help of your affirmations, you can keep your commitments and have plenty of time for a healthy lifestyle.

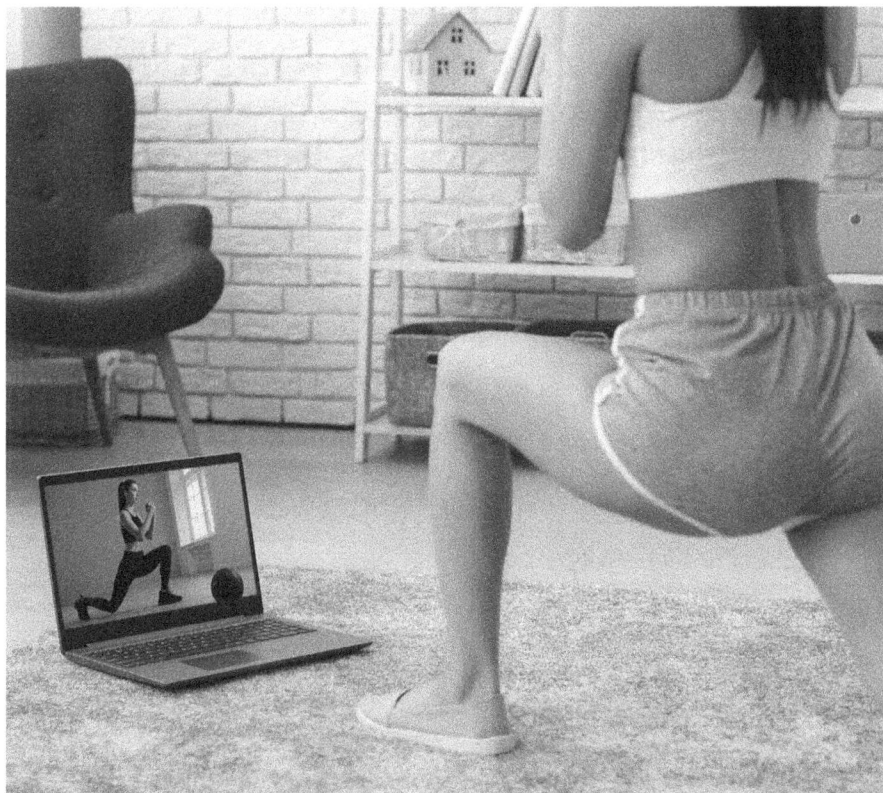

Chapter Six Key Point: Health is a top priority that is crucial for all your other endeavors. You've committed to practice healthy habits, so keep those important appointments with yourself.

Chapter Six Assignment: Evaluate your calendar planning tool(s). Being organized is a mindset, not dependant on any particular device. If the calendar on your smartphone works for you, great. If you would rather use a 79-cent spiral notebook, that's fine, too. Just notice your relationship with the tool you have, and if you're not using it, find something that you WILL use.

Choose one new habit you will commit to doing at least once a week and make an appointment with yourself, blocking out the time in your planner for the next three months. Also, write ideas in your notebook of ways to include new healthy habits with no extra time required.

> **"We cannot put off living until we are ready... it is always urgent, 'here and now,' without any possible postponement. Life is fired at us point-blank."**
>
> **—Jose Ortega y Gasset**

Chapter Seven

Conclusion:
The 10 Secrets for
Maintaining a Healthy Lifestyle

We've almost completed this introduction to the kaizen approach. I want to leave you with 10 crucial secrets that will help you take everything you've learned and use it to effortlessly create your healthy lifestyle.

1. Continually ask the Magic Question: "What's my one next right action?" Remember that kaizen works through small steps for continuous improvement.

2. Write in your healthy lifestyle notebook every day, including positive messages you can refer to for extra motivation down the road.

3. Study your affirmations like they'll be on a big exam. Reading them out loud helps ingrain them—and say it like you mean it! Write new affirmations as the mood strikes you.

4. Track your progress. See Appendix D for examples of Body Metrics Forms.

5. Avoid rushing to try the latest fads, health advice, gimmicks, quick fixes and snake oil.

6. Continue to eliminate tolerations, and check them off your list as you do.

7. Build in plenty of self-rewards along the path. Celebrate the smallest of accomplishments.

8. Schedule active outings and activities. An active lifestyle is a healthy lifestyle.

9. Nurture your healthiest relationships, especially with people also trying to live a healthy lifestyle. Have a Wellness Coach, partner, or exercise buddy keep you accountable.

10. Forgive your negative self-talk and continue to write healthier messages. Rinse and repeat.

Chapter Seven Key Point: There's nothing new in this book. You've heard it all before. What matters is that you've decided to embrace these secrets and utilize these tools to develop and live a life of health and vitality, starting now.

Chapter Seven Assignment: In your healthy lifestyle notebook, write your own healthy tips, kaizen wisdom and inspiration. After all, who is responsible for your health?

"Prayer indeed is good, but while calling on the gods, a man should himself lend a hand."

—Hippocrates

About the Author

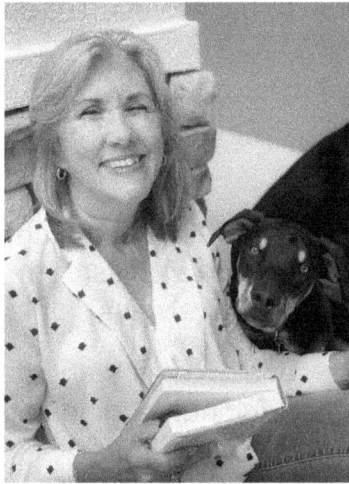

Barbara Dee, MCC

Barbara Dee is an author and speaker, and President of Suncoast Digital Press, Inc. With her B.S. degree in Nutrition Science, Master Certification as a Life Coach, and life-long commitment to well-being, Barbara naturally inspires others to make daily, healthy choices.

She is a magazine columnist and author/publisher of Carpe Diem! and the co-author of *You Can Write A Book! How to Write What You Know and Self-Publish Your Way to Success*. Her popular online course is the Breakthrough Book Master Class, a blueprint for writing any nonfiction book.

Her favorite healthy activity is tarpon fishing.

Connect with Barbara at https://barbara-dee.com/

Mission Statement

My mission is to use my experience and curiosity to distinguish and communicate what Life continuously teaches, to encourage myself and others to discover and strengthen our individual gifts, express them in the world, and contribute to the evolution of appreciation.

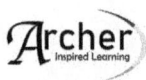

Archer
Inspired Learning

Are you a lifelong learner? Lifelong learning recognizes that not all of our learning comes from a classroom. It is often informal, sometimes free of charge, and always self-initiated.

Whether exploring personal interests and passions or pursuing professional ambitions, lifelong learning can help us to achieve personal fulfillment and satisfaction.

It recognizes that humans have a natural drive to explore, learn, and grow, and encourages us to improve our own quality of life and sense of self-worth by paying attention to the ideas and goals that inspire us.

Yes, make time for learning new things, but also to teach.

Share your lifelong learning, life lessons, your experiences (including the fumbles and game-winners) with others.

We, the committed lifelong learners, are eager to hear what you have to say.

https://www.archerinspiredlearning.com/

Appendices

Appendix A
Tips for Organizing Your Healthy Lifestyle Notebook

Appendix B
How to Create a Purpose-Driven Kitchen

Appendix C
Wheel of Wellness

Appendix D
Utilizing Body Metrics

Appendix E
Ask the Dietitian

Appendix F
Excerpts from the US HHS Guidelines for Americans

Appendix A

Tips for Organizing Your Healthy Lifestyle Notebook

1. **Keep it simple and easy to use**. Don't get fancy or set up something that is no fun to use. Are you more likely to use a spiral notebook or your phone? Do you already have a place where you capture ideas, memorandums, task lists? There is no perfect tool—just the one you will use every day.

2. **Give it a name**. Use motivating and self-friendly words since you will be interacting with this tool every day. Create a title that helps you connect with your desire to be well and enjoy a healthy lifestyle. Examples: My Personal Health Journal; Healthy Notebook; The Kaizen Healthy Lifestyle Notebook; Journal to the Center of My Joy; Feel Good Today; Kaizen Health Diary; Fun, Food and Fitness Journal; Easy Step Healthy Life Guide; Health Notes to Myself; or, Loving Life Journal.

3. **Create categories**. If you are using a notebook, set up different sections with plenty of pages allotted for each section. You may want to try a refillable 3-ring notebook with index dividers. You can expand your notebook as you please with a body metrics chart, healthy recipes, and other sources of inspiration. If you are using a computer or other device, set up your categories, labels or folders, depending on your software or app. Category examples: Old Conversations/Excuses/Limiting Beliefs. Goals and New

Choices. I will... My Wheel of Wellness. Body Metrics Chart. Food Diary. Healthy Staples List. Healthy Travel Checklist. Buddy List (names and contact info of supportive health-minded people). Affirmations. Ideas Which Take No Extra Time. Rewards.

4. **Make a plan to get started**. Where will you keep your notebook? What will remind you to use it every day? How can you add an element of fun (e.g., would you like to use colored pens or pencils)? How private do you need it to be? How can you make it interactive?

5. **Reward yourself just for using your book**. With the kaizen approach, sometimes the first step is the most significant one. Setting up this tool will jumpstart your intentional optimism and using it will definitely help build momentum as you work toward your healthy lifestyle goals. When you don't feel like sticking to any fitness or food plan, write about your resistance in your healthy lifestyle notebook. It gets you into the present moment and can help you recover your motivation. Plan special rewards for using the tool every day for a week, one month, three months, etc. Then claim your reward.

My Total
Wellness
Journal

The Kaizen Method to a Healthy Lifestyle

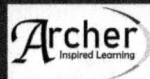

Archer
Inspired Learning

30-Day Health Challenge

START DATE:

THE GOAL: _____

_____

_____

day 1	day 2	day 3	day 4	day 5	day 6	day 7
day 8	day 9	day 10	day 11	day 12	day 13	day 14
day 15	day 16	day 17	day 18	day 19	day 20	day 21
day 22	day 23	day 24	day 25	day 26	day 27	day 28
day 29	day 29					

END DATE:

MY REWARD: _____

_____

The Kaizen Method to a Healthy Lifestyle

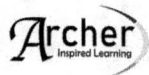

Archer
Inspired Learning

54

Healthy Lifestyle Tracker

Healthy Habits

MONTH: _____

_____
① ② ③ ④ ⑤ ⑥ ⑦ ⑧ ⑨ ⑩ ⑪ ⑫ ⑬ ⑭ ⑮
⑯ ⑰ ⑱ ⑲ ⑳ ㉑ ㉒ ㉓ ㉔ ㉕ ㉖ ㉗ ㉘ ㉙ ㉚

_____
① ② ③ ④ ⑤ ⑥ ⑦ ⑧ ⑨ ⑩ ⑪ ⑫ ⑬ ⑭ ⑮
⑯ ⑰ ⑱ ⑲ ⑳ ㉑ ㉒ ㉓ ㉔ ㉕ ㉖ ㉗ ㉘ ㉙ ㉚

_____
① ② ③ ④ ⑤ ⑥ ⑦ ⑧ ⑨ ⑩ ⑪ ⑫ ⑬ ⑭ ⑮
⑯ ⑰ ⑱ ⑲ ⑳ ㉑ ㉒ ㉓ ㉔ ㉕ ㉖ ㉗ ㉘ ㉙ ㉚

_____
① ② ③ ④ ⑤ ⑥ ⑦ ⑧ ⑨ ⑩ ⑪ ⑫ ⑬ ⑭ ⑮
⑯ ⑰ ⑱ ⑲ ⑳ ㉑ ㉒ ㉓ ㉔ ㉕ ㉖ ㉗ ㉘ ㉙ ㉚

_____
① ② ③ ④ ⑤ ⑥ ⑦ ⑧ ⑨ ⑩ ⑪ ⑫ ⑬ ⑭ ⑮
⑯ ⑰ ⑱ ⑲ ⑳ ㉑ ㉒ ㉓ ㉔ ㉕ ㉖ ㉗ ㉘ ㉙ ㉚

_____
① ② ③ ④ ⑤ ⑥ ⑦ ⑧ ⑨ ⑩ ⑪ ⑫ ⑬ ⑭ ⑮
⑯ ⑰ ⑱ ⑲ ⑳ ㉑ ㉒ ㉓ ㉔ ㉕ ㉖ ㉗ ㉘ ㉙ ㉚

_____
① ② ③ ④ ⑤ ⑥ ⑦ ⑧ ⑨ ⑩ ⑪ ⑫ ⑬ ⑭ ⑮
⑯ ⑰ ⑱ ⑲ ⑳ ㉑ ㉒ ㉓ ㉔ ㉕ ㉖ ㉗ ㉘ ㉙ ㉚

_____
① ② ③ ④ ⑤ ⑥ ⑦ ⑧ ⑨ ⑩ ⑪ ⑫ ⑬ ⑭ ⑮
⑯ ⑰ ⑱ ⑲ ⑳ ㉑ ㉒ ㉓ ㉔ ㉕ ㉖ ㉗ ㉘ ㉙ ㉚

_____
① ② ③ ④ ⑤ ⑥ ⑦ ⑧ ⑨ ⑩ ⑪ ⑫ ⑬ ⑭ ⑮
⑯ ⑰ ⑱ ⑲ ⑳ ㉑ ㉒ ㉓ ㉔ ㉕ ㉖ ㉗ ㉘ ㉙ ㉚

The Kaizen Method to a Healthy Lifestyle

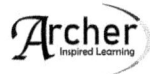

Archer
Inspired Learning

My GET ACTIVE Plan

MONTH:						
SUN	MON	TUES	WED	THUR	FRI	SAT

NOTES

The Kaizen Method to a Healthy Lifestyle

Archer
Inspired Learning

Healthy Eating Plan

	BREAKFAST	LIUNCH	DINNER	SNACKS
MON				
TUES				
WED				
THURS				
FRI				
SAT				
SUN				

The Kaizen Method to a Healthy Lifestyle

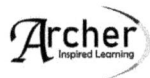

Archer
Inspired Learning

57

A Thoughtful Grocery List

CATEGORY:

☐ _____

☐ _____

☐ _____

☐ _____

☐ _____

☐ _____

☐ _____

CATEGORY:

☐ _____

☐ _____

☐ _____

☐ _____

☐ _____

☐ _____

☐ _____

The Kaizen Method to a Healthy Lifestyle

Archer
Inspired Learning

My Activities and Exercise

Activity and Measure:_____

Activity and Measure:_____

Activity and Measure:_____

Activity and Measure:_____

Activity and Measure:_____

Activity and Measure:_____

Activity and Measure:_____

Activity and Measure:_____

Activity and Measure:_____

Activity and Measure:_____

NOTES

The Kaizen Method to a Healthy Lifestyle

Archer
Inspired Learning

My Health Improves One Day at a Time

DATE: _____

S   M   T   W   T   F   S

TODAY'S SCHEDULE

7AM

8AM

9AM

10AM

11AM

12AM

1PM

2PM

3PM

4PM

5PM

6PM

7PM

HEALTHY FOCUS AREA

1. _____ ☐

2. _____ ☐

3. _____ ☐

4. _____ ☐

5. _____ ☐

MEALS

BREAKFAST

LUNCH

DINNER

SNACKS

The Kaizen Method to a Healthy Lifestyle

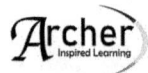

Archer Inspired Learning

60

My Health Improves One Week at a Time

WEEK OF:_____

MONDAY

TUESDAY

WEDNESDAY

THURSDAY

FRIDAY

SATURDAY

SUNDAY

HEALTHY FOCUS AREA

1. _____ ☐

2 _____ ☐

3 _____ ☐

4 _____ ☐

5. _____ ☐

FOR NEXT WEEK

NOTES

The Kaizen Method to a Healthy Lifestyle

Archer
Inspired Learning

My Food Diary

MON

DATE_____

calorie goal

calorie actual

TODAY'S MEALS:

BREAKFAST:

LUNCH:

DINNER:

SNACKS:

The Kaizen Method to a Healthy Lifestyle

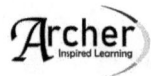

Archer Inspired Learning

62

My Active Lifestyle

WHY DO YOU WANT TO BE MORE ACTIVE AND FIT?

Fitness goes beyond the physical. Having important and personal reasons for fitness is important.

WHAT ARE THE BENEFITS OF AN ACTIVE LIFESTYLE?

What benefits do you anticipate from adopting an active lifestyle?

WHAT ARE THE OBSTACLES OF BEING ACTIVE EVERY DAY?

What obstacles do you anticipate from adopting a daily active focus?

The Kaizen Method to a Healthy Lifestyle

Archer
Inspired Learning

My Active Lifestyle

HOW WILL YOU OVERCOME OBSTACLES?

Describe the ways you will conquer the fitness obstacles you will face.

WHERE DO YOU SEE YOURSELF ONE YEAR FROM NOW?

Briefly describe where you see yourself on your fitness journey a year from now? Describe your physical status and mental outlook.

WHAT WILL YOU NEED IN YOUR LIFE TO ACHIEVE YOUR ACTIVE LIFESTYLE GOALS?

List at least 5 ways you will have built-in reinforcement and support. (Friends, family, healthy lifestyle journal, fitness apps, health coach, etc.)

The Kaizen Method to a Healthy Lifestyle

Archer
Inspired Learning

Healthy Eating Worksheet

HOW DO YOU DEFINE HEALTHY EATING?
Healthy Eating starts with being mindful. What do you want to be mindful of?

WHAT ARE THE BENEFITS OF HEALTHY EATING?
What benefits do you anticipate from more mindful, healthy eating?

WHAT OBSTACLES WILL YOU FACE WITH HEALTHY EATING?
Describe the obstacles you anticipate from being more mindful about healthy eating.

The Kaizen Method to a Healthy Lifestyle

Archer
Inspired Learning

Healthy Eating Worksheet

HOW WILL YOU OVERCOME YOUR HEALTHY EATING OBSTACLES?

List ways to overcome the obstacles you anticipate to your new healthy eating lifestyle.

WHAT KIND OF SUPPORT WILL HELP YOU WITH MORE MINDFUL, HEALTHY EATING?

Will you need support from friends and family? New recipes, apps, cookbooks, or cooking classes? Describe in detail what support you will need for more healthier, mindful eating.

WHERE DO YOU SEE YOURSELF IN THE FUTURE?

Write a description of a healthier you six months, and one year from now. Standing in your healthier self's future, how has healthier eating impacted your life in a positive way? How have your new eating habits impacted those closest to you?

The Kaizen Method to a Healthy Lifestyle

Archer
Inspired Learning

66

Favorite Healthy Foods and Meals
~Breakfast and Lunch~

This is my helpful reminder page. There really are many things I like to eat which are nutritious, too! I will choose from these:

MY FAVORITE HEALTHY
BREAKFAST FOODS

HEALTHY BREAKFAST
MEALS

MY FAVORITE HEALTHY
LUNCH FOODS

HEALTHY LUNCH
MEALS

The Kaizen Method to a Healthy Lifestyle

Favorite Healthy Foods and Meals
~Dinner and Snacks~

**MY FAVORITE HEALTHY
DINNER FOODS**

HEALTHY DINNER MEALS

**MY FAVORITE HEALTHY
SNACK FOODS**

MY FAVORITE ZERO-SUGAR DRINKS

The Kaizen Method to a Healthy Lifestyle

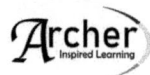

Archer Inspired Learning

Why My Healthy Lifestyle Matters

_____
_____
_____
_____
_____
_____
_____
_____
_____
_____
_____
_____
_____
_____
_____
_____
_____
_____
_____
_____
_____
_____
_____
_____

The Kaizen Method to a Healthy Lifestyle

Ideas for New Activities to Try

Ideas for New Healthy Foods or Recipes to Try

Sample Notebook Pages in Use

Following are examples of healthy lifestyle notebook pages in use. Select the forms, format, and focus that are the best match for you and your health goals.

Using a spiral notebook with no forms is fine, too. Whatever serves your purpose and makes you want to utilize it every day is perfect.

Healthy Lifestyle Tracker

Healthy Habits MONTH: _October_

(8) waters 8 oz each
⑨ ⑩ ⑪ ⑫ ⑬ ⑭ ⑮
⑯ ⑰ ⑱ ⑲ ⑳ ㉑ ㉒ ㉓ ㉔ ㉕ ㉖ ㉗ ㉘ ㉙ ㉚

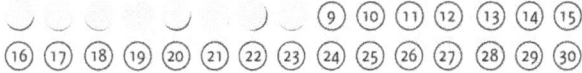

keep food dairy
⑨ ⑩ ⑪ ⑫ ⑬ ⑭ ⑮
⑯ ⑰ ⑱ ⑲ ⑳ ㉑ ㉒ ㉓ ㉔ ㉕ ㉖ ㉗ ㉘ ㉙ ㉚

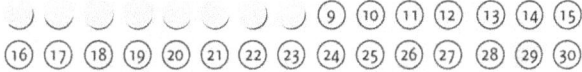

20 min neck & back stretch
⑤ ⑥ ⑨ ⑩ ⑪ ⑫ ⑬ ⑭ ⑮
⑯ ⑰ ⑱ ⑲ ⑳ ㉑ ㉒ ㉓ ㉔ ㉕ ㉖ ㉗ ㉘ ㉙ ㉚

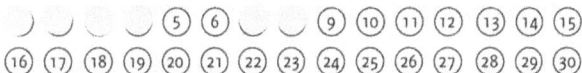

30 min walk with meditation app
② ④ ⑥ ⑧ ⑨ ⑩ ⑪ ⑫ ⑬ ⑭ ⑮
⑯ ⑰ ⑱ ⑲ ⑳ ㉑ ㉒ ㉓ ㉔ ㉕ ㉖ ㉗ ㉘ ㉙ ㉚

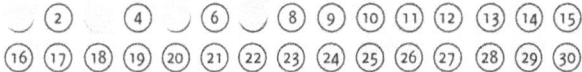

review healthy lifestyle journal
③ ④ ⑦ ⑧ ⑨ ⑩ ⑪ ⑫ ⑬ ⑭ ⑮
⑯ ⑰ ⑱ ⑲ ⑳ ㉑ ㉒ ㉓ ㉔ ㉕ ㉖ ㉗ ㉘ ㉙ ㉚

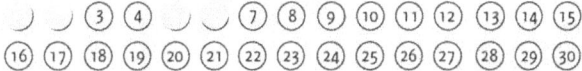

sleep- go to bed by 10
④ ⑧ ⑨ ⑩ ⑪ ⑫ ⑬ ⑭ ⑮
⑯ ⑰ ⑱ ⑲ ⑳ ㉑ ㉒ ㉓ ㉔ ㉕ ㉖ ㉗ ㉘ ㉙ ㉚

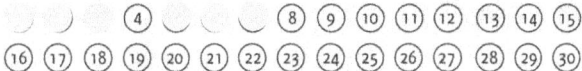

take Vitamin D and zinc
⑨ ⑩ ⑪ ⑫ ⑬ ⑭ ⑮
⑯ ⑰ ⑱ ⑲ ⑳ ㉑ ㉒ ㉓ ㉔ ㉕ ㉖ ㉗ ㉘ ㉙ ㉚

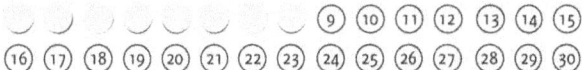

25 reps with hand weights
② ④ ⑥ ⑧ ⑨ ⑩ ⑪ ⑫ ⑬ ⑭ ⑮
⑯ ⑰ ⑱ ⑲ ⑳ ㉑ ㉒ ㉓ ㉔ ㉕ ㉖ ㉗ ㉘ ㉙ ㉚

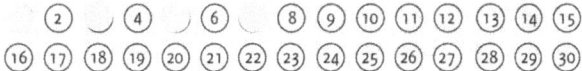

do yoga with video (15 min)
① ③ ⑤ ⑦ ⑨ ⑩ ⑪ ⑫ ⑬ ⑭ ⑮
⑯ ⑰ ⑱ ⑲ ⑳ ㉑ ㉒ ㉓ ㉔ ㉕ ㉖ ㉗ ㉘ ㉙ ㉚

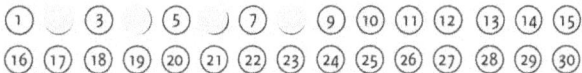

The Kaizen Method to a Healthy Lifestyle Archer Inspired Learning

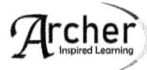

My GET ACTIVE Plan

MONTH: *October*

SUN	MON	TUES	WED	THUR	FRI	SAT
				1 bike-65 min	**2** walk-20 min. 45 min	**3** walk-60 min
4 bike-45 min	**5** walk & fish 90 min	**6** walk- 15 min. 50 min	**7** walk- 15 min 45 min	**8** bike- 60 min	**9**	**10**
11	**12**	**13**	**14**	**15**	**16**	**17**
18	**19**	**20**	**21**	**22**	**23**	**24**
25	**26**	**27**	**28**	**29**	**30**	**31**

NOTES

I will be active and move my body every day. My goal is to walk or bike or kayak or a combo of activities for at least one hour, total time.

The Kaizen Method to a Healthy Lifestyle

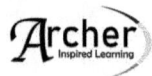

Archer
Inspired Learning

74

A Thoughtful Grocery List

CATEGORY: *Fruits & veggies*

- [ ] apples
- [ ] avocados
- [ ] bell pepper
- [ ] kiwi
- [ ] roma tomatoes
- [ ] _____
- [ ] _____

CATEGORY: *Protein*

- [ ] organic chicken breasts
- [ ] grass-fed ground beef
- [ ] frozen cod fillets
- [ ] wild caught salmon
- [ ] _____
- [ ] _____
- [ ] _____

The Kaizen Method to a Healthy Lifestyle

Archer
Inspired Learning

This is my helpful reminder page. There really are many things I like to eat which are nutritious, too! I will choose from these:

MY FAVORITE HEALTHY BREAKFAST FOODS

--avocado
--pears
--strawberry yogurt
--blueberries
--plain yogurt
--walnuts
--poached eggs
--Swiss cheese

HEALTHY BREAKFAST MEALS

--Avocado toast
--2 poached eggs on 1 pc toast
--scrambled eggs with Swiss, bell pepper, and onion
--plain yogurt with tsp honey and walnuts
--strawberry smoothie with whey protein powder and almond milk

MY FAVORITE HEALTHY LUNCH FOODS

--turkey slices
--avocado
--hard-boiled egg
--Swiss cheese
--rye toast
--tomato

HEALTHY LUNCH MEALS

-grilled Swiss (1 pc toast) with tomato
-hard-boiled egg and olives
-smoothie with almond milk and whey protein
-turkey slices with mustard
-toast with almond butter and blueberries

The Kaizen Method to a Healthy Lifestyle

Archer
Inspired Learning

Ideas for New Healthy Foods or Recipes to Try

Cornish hen

Moroccan grilled chicken (ask Dara)

Baked tomatoes with basil and parm

Spicy yogurt dressing (ask Ava)

Asian pear salad

Edamame salad

Cumin gravy for turkey

Zucchini crab cakes

Mango and hot pepper relish

Shrimp and squash kabobs (ask Deb)

Appendix B

How to Create a Purpose-Driven Kitchen

Every room in your home has a purpose. If your home is a reflection of who you are, then your kitchen is a reflection of the way you eat and the role of food in your life. You are responsible for intentionally setting up your environment to support your healthy lifestyle, and your kitchen is an excellent place to start. More than simply a convenient place to store and prepare food, your kitchen can serve a higher purpose as a center for nourishment and a partner in your healthy lifestyle.

What are three common mistakes that can turn your kitchen against you?

1. **Unhealthy foods on hand**. Processed, high-calorie/low nutritive value foods do not fit into your healthy lifestyle. If others in your household insist on stocking junk, confine it to a certain cabinet or shelf and make sure it's behind closed doors. Always shop with a list so you are making wise choices and not bringing home impulse purchases out of old habit.

2. **Placement without priority**. Give your healthiest foods top priority for easy accessibility and visibility. Make it easy to make good choices. If you want to increase your servings of fresh fruit or amount of water you drink, keep these priority choices visible and handy.

3. **Clutter**. Confusion and clutter detract from your high-level priority of healthy eating. Whether it's mail, homework, bills or dirty dishes, keep the clutter away so you can have a peaceful mind as you nourish your body. Additionally, it's a good idea to reevaluate your inventory of small appliances and kitchen-aids. Toss the Fry-Daddy, for example.

By addressing these issues, you can create a kitchen where you can avoid temptations, reach for convenient healthy choices, and find a comfortable place to practice conscious meal planning and healthy cooking.

A purpose-driven kitchen encourages you to stay motivated, and supports you as you rediscover your taste for natural foods. A purpose-driven kitchen saves you money—you plan ahead and purchase wisely. There is always an abundance of healthy food choices—no more desperate calls for pizza delivery just because your cupboard is bare.

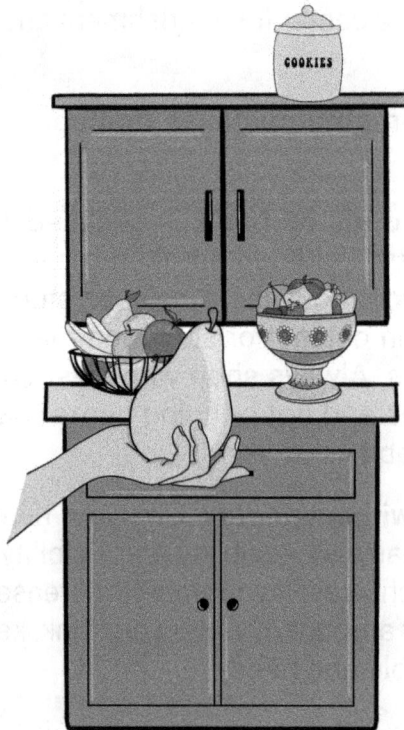

Easy steps to have a purpose-driven kitchen:

1. Take one small area at a time and go through every item deciding if it's the good, the bad or the ugly. You will eventually clean out and reorganize your pantry, snack basket/shelf, spices and seasonings, drawers, cabinets, refrigerator, freezer and supplies.

2. Create a "Healthy Staples" checklist. What makes sense to have on hand at all times? My healthy staples include whole-grain crackers, Greek yogurt, stevia sweetener, black beans, healthy frozen entrées, and almond milk, protein powder and frozen berries for smoothies. You can also include healthy staples for when you are away from your home kitchen—walnuts for the car, a protein bar for your purse, yogurt for the fridge at work, or apples for your travel bag. As you use up these items, add them to your weekly grocery list.

3. Begin a list of your favorite home-prepared healthy meals. As you build that repertoire it will become easier and easier to plan meals for the week, make a shopping list, and purchase just what you need. One easy system is to list a whole meal on the front of a 5x7 card and all the ingredients required for the recipes and preparation on the back. Then you can choose the meal, and easily check to see what you have or what goes on the shopping list.

When you enter your purpose-driven kitchen, you will be inspired to stay true to yourself, and to your new healthy lifestyle habits.

Appendix C

Wheel of Wellness

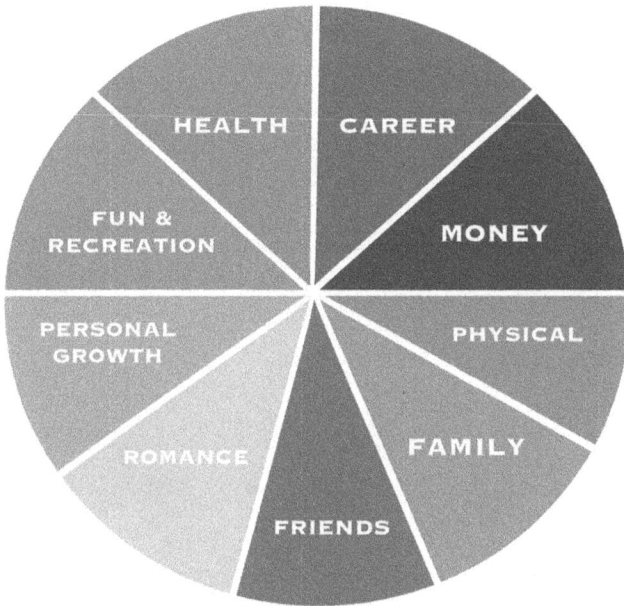

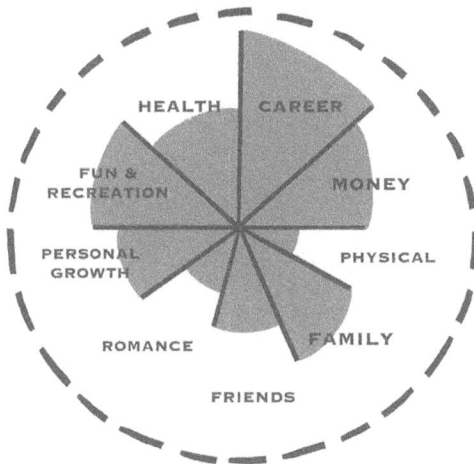

Optimum wellness in each area will even out your wheel, then life will be a smooth ride!

Appendix D

Utilizing Body Metrics

Why Measure? It's been proven that the practice of tracking body measurements accelerates results. It is, however, important to find the optimum period of time between measuring which feels right to you and helps you stay on track and motivated. No one should weigh themselves every day, for example, because your weight could be up or down 1-3 pounds due to many variables; therefore, you are not getting an accurate account of weight loss or weight gain progress. Once a week or even once a month may be the best plan for you—just be sure you use the same scale, around the same time of day, and record the date and result on a Body Metrics Form, paper or electronic version.

If you frequent a gym, have a trainer assist you. Most facilities will have a special scale or way to measure % Body Fat, BMI, visceral fat and heart rate. You will also want to use a tape measure to record waist, arm, hips and thigh measurements periodically. Or you can purchase various body metric devices to have at home. Just decide what you want to track. It could be as simple as wearing a pedometer to count your steps each day. Building up to 10,000 steps a day is an example of a great healthy lifestyle goal for most people. Body Media FIT is an arm band you wear which has skin sensors measuring activity level, calories burned, amount of sleep and so forth, then sends the data to your smart phone for you to see and keep track. There is no one perfect tool for tracking body metrics, only the one you will consistently use.

EXAMPLE: Mike's Body Metrics Form tracking 9 measurable results. (YOU choose what to track.)

Date	Weight	%Body Fat	BMI	Visceral Fat	Chest	Arm	Waist	Thigh

EXAMPLE: Jill's Body Metrics Form tracking 3 measurable results. (YOU choose what to track.)

	Mon	Tue	Wed	Thurs	Fri	Sat	Sun
Steps							
Water							
Weight							

Note: 'Steps' are measured by a pedometer which she doesn't wear on Sundays. 'Water' is to help her develop the habit of drinking 8 glasses a day. 'Weight' is only noted once a week.

Appendix E

Ask the Dietitian

**25 Tips When You Want the Habit of Eating Less
And Still Enjoy Satisfying Meals and Eating Out**

1. At home, after serving your plate, cover the extra food and put it away before you sit down to eat.

2. Divide extra food into single portions before putting it into the refrigerator or freezer.

3. Read "Serving Size" first on a food label.

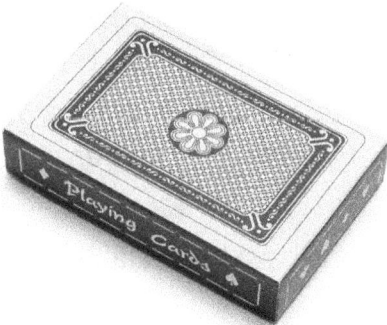

One 3 oz. serving of meat, fish or poultry is the size of a a deck of cards.

4. Use a kitchen scale to weigh foods until you know what a portion looks like.

5. Use a smaller dinner plate.

6. Cancel your membership in the "Clean Plate Club."

7. Make zip-lock snack bags with <100 cal. each using almonds, craisins, lo-cal popcorn, etc. Use at home, at your office, or grab-and-go.

8. Write 100 times: Better to Waste than Add It To My Waist.

9. Calculate amount of exercise required to burn those extra calories you are considering and ask yourself if you will do that exercise within 90 minutes.

10. Eat the highest fiber foods on your plate first—vegetables, beans, wild rice, etc.

11. Eat a protein shake or snack before you go out to dinner.

12. Do not open the menu. You know the restaurant or type of food well enough to decide on a healthy meal to order. Inside the menu are land mines—color photos of mac-n-cheese, item after item you rather not consume, and psychologically masterminded descriptions of huge desserts. The key to guilt-free dining out is to get through the 45 seconds it takes to talk with the server and decide what to order. Then you can relax!

13. Sometimes you can order an appetizer rather than an entrée (save money and calories!)

14. Order one entre for two people and have the restaurant split it before serving.

15. Ask for To-Go box when the server brings your meal—go ahead and put half your meal in it.

16. Keep a food diary! Write down every single calorie you eat for 5 days. (See examples in Appendix A.) You may be shocked at how less mindful you have been than you realized.

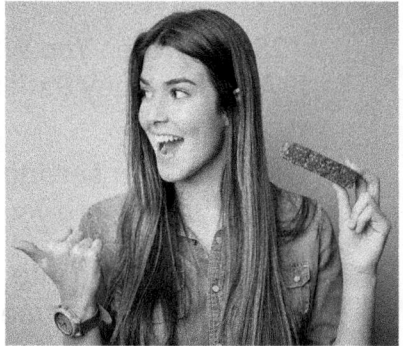

17. Slow down. Count 25 chews per bite to foster the habit of eating more slowly, or use your opposite hand to hold the fork to slow down your eating. Or put down your fork between bites.

18. Use the paper napkin trick. (If you take a bite and it's not delicious—put a napkin to your mouth and let those calories go into the napkin instead of into your body. Never swallow something just to get it out of your mouth or away from your taste buds.)

19. Drink 8 oz. of water, green tea, broth, or diet club soda just before your meal.

20. Do not eat in front of the TV or while reading. Your brain is too distracted to realize how much you are eating. Stay as mindful as possible and savor your food. Practice describing the tastes.

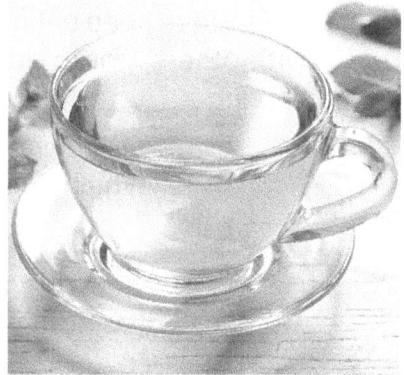

21. Add as much spice as you can to your food. Strong Indian spices, for example, curb the appetite.

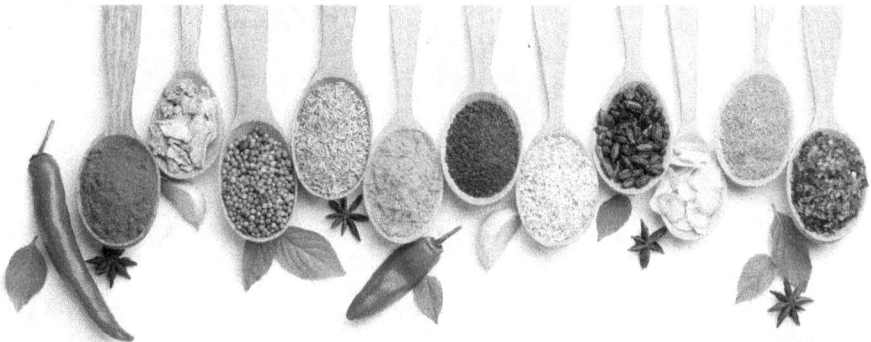

22. To help you slow down, plan to tell an amusing story at the table and start it after you've had 25% of your meal.

23. Survey the entire buffet bar before starting through the line. You will then know what you have decided to put on your plate before you start.

24. Eat half your lunch at noon and the other half at 3 p.m. (When you keep your blood sugar levels more even, you won't feel tired or hungry.)

25. Carry sugarless peppermint gum or mints and put in your mouth as soon as you've had enough to eat. You won't be tempted to keep eating just because you're still at the table with others, nor to order a dessert just to satisfy a sweet craving.

Which tip will you try today?

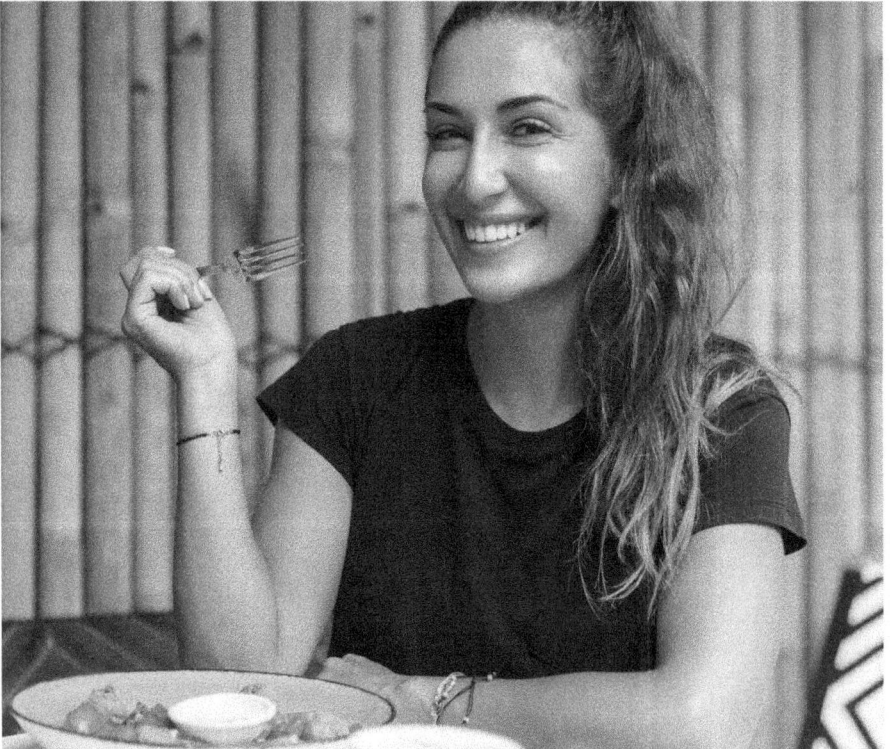

Appendix F

Excerpts from the US Department of Health and Human Services

Guidelines for Americans

The 2018 *Physical Activity Guidelines Advisory Committee Scientific Report* provided the content and conceptual underpinning for the Guidelines. Key elements of this framework are described in the following sections.

Disease Prevention and Health Promotion

The 2008 Advisory Committee Report and the 2008 Guidelines focused primarily on the disease prevention benefits of physical activity.

The 2018 Scientific Report demonstrates that, in addition to disease prevention benefits, regular physical activity provides a variety of other benefits, including helping people sleep better, feel better, and perform daily tasks more easily. The 2018 Scientific Report also notes immediate benefits of physical activity in addition to those related to regular physical activity over months or years. This broader focus on both disease prevention and health promotion is embedded in the key guidelines for the amounts and types of physical activity that are provided for three age groups (children and adolescents, adults, and older adults), for women who are pregnant or postpartum, and for adults with chronic diseases or adults with disabilities.

Strong evidence demonstrates that moderate-to-vigorous physical activity improves the quality of sleep in adults. It does so by reducing the length of time it takes to go to sleep and reducing the time one is awake after going to sleep and before rising in the morning. It also can increase the time in deep sleep and reduce daytime sleepiness.

Strong evidence from adults demonstrates that perceived quality of life is improved by regular physical activity. The Guidelines focuses on selected aspects of health-related quality of life, including both physical and mental or emotional health. It does not include other aspects of quality of life, such as those related to finances, relationships, or occupations.

Physical activity improves physical function among individuals of all ages, enabling them to conduct their daily lives with energy and without undue fatigue. This is true for older adults, for whom improved physical function reduces risk of falls and fall-related injuries and contributes to their ability to maintain independence. It is also true for young and middle-aged adults, as improved physical function helps them more easily accomplish the tasks of daily living, such as climbing stairs or carrying groceries.

In addition to improving physical function, physical activity may improve cognitive function among youth and adults. Aspects of cognitive function that may be improved include memory, attention, executive function (the ability to plan and organize; monitor, inhibit, or facilitate behaviors; initiate tasks; and control emotions), and academic performance among youth.

Timing of Benefits

A single session of moderate-to-vigorous physical activity can reduce blood pressure, improve insulin sensitivity, improve sleep, reduce anxiety symptoms, and improve some aspects of cognition on the day that it is performed. Most of these improvements become even larger with the regular performance of moderate-to-vigorous physical activity. Other benefits, such as disease risk reduction and improved physical function, accrue within days to weeks after consistently being more physically active.

Physical Activity Intensity

The Guidelines consider the intensity with which people do physical activity. Some activities are a higher intensity than others because they require more energy to do. For example, a person expends more energy walking briskly than slowly strolling.

Absolute rates of energy expenditure during physical activity are commonly described as light, moderate, or vigorous intensity. Energy expenditure is expressed by multiples of the metabolic equivalent of task (MET), where 1 MET is the rate of energy expenditure while sitting at rest.

- ▶ Light-intensity activity is non-sedentary waking behavior that requires less than 3.0 METs; examples include walking at a slow or leisurely pace (2 mph or less), cooking activities, or light household chores.

- ▶ Moderate-intensity activity requires 3.0 to less than 6.0 METs; examples include walking briskly (2.5 to 4 mph), playing doubles tennis, or raking the yard.

- ▶ Vigorous-intensity activity requires 6.0 or more METs; examples include jogging, running, carrying heavy groceries or other loads upstairs, shoveling snow, or participating in a strenuous fitness class. Many adults do no vigorous-intensity physical activity.

Levels of Physical Activity

Throughout the Guidelines, reference is made to four levels of aerobic physical activity: inactive, insufficiently active, active, and highly active. This classification for adults is useful because these categories are related to how much health benefit a person obtains at a given level and how to become more active.

The focus on aerobic physical activity for the levels should not be interpreted to suggest that other types of activity, such as muscle strengthening, are less important.

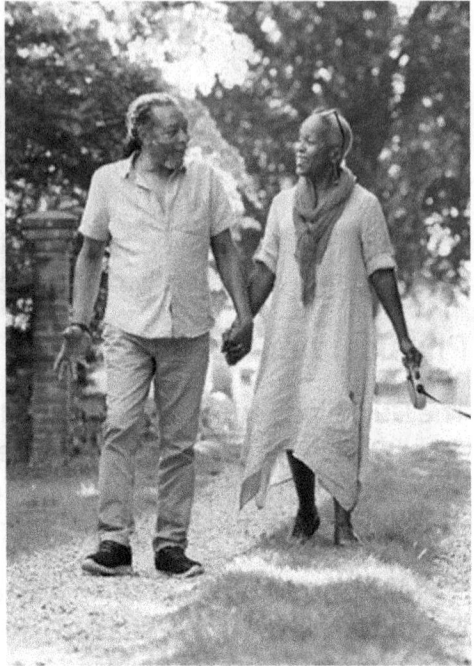

▸ **Inactive** is not getting any moderate- or vigorous-intensity physical activity beyond basic movement from daily life activities.

▸ **Insufficiently active** is doing some moderate- or vigorous-intensity physical activity but less than 150minutes of moderate-intensity physical activity a week or 75 minutes of vigorous-intensity physical activity or the equivalent combination. This level is less than the target range for meeting the key guidelines for adults.

▸ **Active** is doing the equivalent of 150 minutes to 300 minutes of moderate-intensity physical activity a week. This level meets the key guideline target range for adults.

Highly active is doing the equivalent of more than 300 minutes of moderate-intensity physical activity a week. This level exceeds the key guideline target range for adults.

The Relationship Between Sedentary Behavior and Physical Activity

Research on the health effects of sedentary behavior is a relatively new area. Therefore, it was not addressed in 2008. Sedentary behavior has received an increasing amount of attention as a public health problem because it appears to have health risks, and it is a highly prevalent behavior in the U.S. population. Data collected by devices in the U.S. National Health and Nutrition Examination Survey (NHANES) indicate that children and adults spend approximately 7.7 hours per day (55% of their monitored waking time) being sedentary. Thus, the potential population health impact of sedentary behavior is substantial.

The 2018 Advisory Committee found a strong relationship between time in sedentary behavior and the risk of all-cause mortality and cardiovascular disease mortality in adults. However, the literature was insufficient to recommend a specific target for adults or youth for how many times during the day sedentary time should be interrupted with physical activity. Furthermore, a specific healthy target for total sedentary behavior time could not be determined. This was because the risk related to sedentary behavior was dependent upon the amount of moderate-to-vigorous physical activity performed.

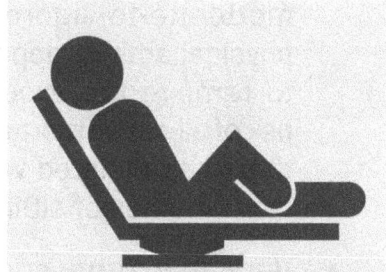

What Is Sedentary Behavior?

In general, sedentary behavior refers to any waking behavior characterized by a low level of energy expenditure (less than or equal to 1.5 METs) while sitting, reclining, or lying. The Guidelines operationalizes the definition of sedentary behavior to include self-reported sitting (leisure-time, occupational, and total), television (TV) viewing or screen time, and low levels of movement measured by devices that assess movement or posture. Standing is another activity with low energy expenditure, but it is distinct from sedentary behavior in how it affects health.

95

Three main conclusions:

▶ High volumes of moderate-to-vigorous physical activity appear to remove the excess risk of all-cause mortality that is associated with high volumes of sitting.

▶ Very low time spent sitting reduces, but does not eliminate, the risk of no moderate-to-vigorous physical activity.

▶ Given the high levels of sitting and low levels of physical activity in the population, most people would benefit from both increasing moderate-to-vigorous physical activity and reducing time spent sitting.

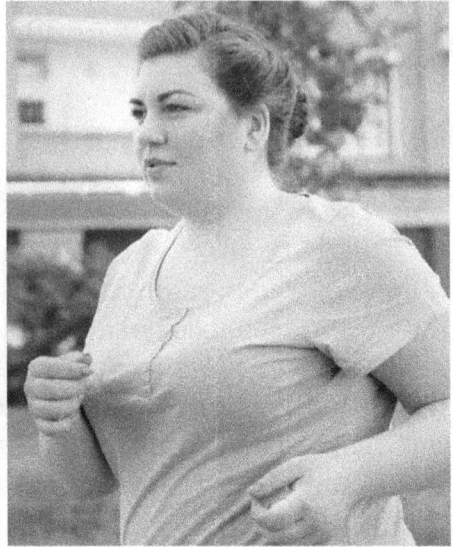

Progressing Toward and Beyond the Physical Activity Target

The 2008 Advisory Committee reported that inactive people can achieve substantial health gains by increasing their activity level even if they do not reach the target range. Since 2008, substantially more information documents the value of reducing inactivity even if youth or adults do not achieve the recommended target range.

Bouts, or episodes, of moderate-to-vigorous physical activity of any duration may be included in the daily accumulated total volume of physical activity. The 2008 Physical Activity Guidelines for Americans recommended accumulating moderate-to-vigorous physical activity in bouts of 10 minutes or more because not enough evidence was available to support the value of bouts less than 10 minutes in duration. The 2018 Advisory Committee concluded that bouts of any length contribute to the health benefits associated with the accumulated volume of physical activity. Even a brief episode of physical activity like climbing up a few flights of stairs counts.

Bouts of any length contribute to the health benefits associated with the accumulated volume of physical activity.

What Does "Progressing Toward Targets" Mean for People's Daily Lives?

The risk of injury to bones, muscles, and joints is directly related to the gap between a person's usual level of activity and a new level of activity. When amounts of physical activity need to be increased to meet the key guidelines or personal goals, physical activity should be increased gradually over time, no matter what the person's current level of physical activity.

For people who are inactive, that is, people who do not do any moderate- or vigorous-intensity physical activity beyond basic movement from daily life activities:

- ▸ Reducing sedentary behavior has health benefits. It reduces the risk of all-cause mortality, cardiovasculardisease incidence and mortality, and the incidence of type 2 diabetes and some cancers. A good firststep is to replace sedentary behavior with light-intensity physical activity. Previously, evidence that light-intensity physical activity could provide health benefits was not sufficient to support a recommendation.

- ▸ No matter how much time they spend in sedentary behavior or light-intensity activity, inactive peoplecan reduce their health risks by gradually increasing their moderate-intensity physical activity.

For people who are insufficiently active, that is, people who do some moderate- or vigorous-intensity physical activity, but who do not yet meet the key guidelines target range (150 to 300 minutes a week of moderate-intensity physical activity for adults):

- ▸ Even small increases in moderate-intensity physical activity provide health benefits. There is nothreshold that must be exceeded before benefits begin to occur.

▶ Greater benefits can be achieved by reducing sedentary behavior, increasing moderate-intensityphysical activity, or a combination of both.

▶ For any given increase in moderate-to-vigorous physical activity, the relative gain in benefits is greaterfor insufficiently active people than for people who are already meeting the key guidelines.

For people who are active, that is, people who already meet the key guidelines (150 to 300 minutes a week of moderate-intensity physical activity for adults):

▶ Although those within the target range already have substantial benefits from their current volume ofphysical activity, more benefits can be gained by doing additional moderate-to-vigorous physical activityor reducing sedentary behavior.

For people who are highly active, that is, people who do more than the equivalent of 300 minutes a week of moderate-intensity physical activity:

▶ These people should maintain or increase their activity level by doing a variety of activities.

Health Benefits Versus Other Reasons to Be Physically Active

Although the Guidelines focuses on the health benefits of physical activity, these benefits are not the only reason why people are active. Physical activity gives people a chance to have fun, be with friends and family, enjoy the outdoors, and improve fitness so they can more easily participate in additional physical activity or sporting events. Some people are active because it helps them feel more energetic and healthier.

Nothing in the Guidelines is intended to mean that health benefits are the only reason to do physical activity. People should be physically active for any and all reasons that are meaningful for them.

Health-Related Versus Performance-Related Fitness

Promoting health, reducing risk of chronic disease, and promoting health-related fitness—particularly cardiovascular and muscular fitness—are the primary focus of the Guidelines. People can gain this kind of fitness by doing the amounts and types of activities recommended in the key guidelines for each age group and population.

The types and amounts of activity necessary to improve performance-related fitness are not addressed in the Guidelines. Athletes need this kind of fitness when they compete. Medical screening issues for competitive athletes also are outside the scope of the Guidelines.

People who are interested in training programs to increase performance-related fitness should seek advice from other sources. Generally, these people do much more activity than required to meet the targets in the key guidelines.

Lifespan Approach

The best way to be physically active is to be active for life. Therefore, the Guidelines takes a lifespan approach and provides recommendations for three broad age groups—children and adolescents, adults, and older adults.

The 2008 Guidelines provided recommendations for children, adolescents, and adults, covering individuals ages 6 years and older. Recent research has provided support for recommendations for children ages 3 through 5 years, and so the 2018 Guidelines are designed for those ages 3 years and older. Physical activity is necessary for healthy growth and development of infants and young children of all ages.

Putting the Guidelines Into Practice

Assessing Whether Physical Activity Programs Are Consistent With the Guidelines

Programs that provide opportunities for physical activity, such as classes or community activities, can help people meet the key guidelines. These programs do not have to provide all, or even most, of the recommended weekly activity. For example, a mall walking program for older adults may meet only once a week yet provide useful amounts of activity, as long as people get the rest of their weekly recommended activity on other days.

Programs that are consistent with the Physical Activity Guidelines for Americans:

- ▶ Provide advice and education consistent with the Guidelines;

- ▶ Add episodes of activity that count toward meeting the key guidelines; and

- ▶ May also include activities, such as stretching or warming up and cooling down, whose health benefitsare not yet proven but that are often used in effective physical activity programs.

All Americans should engage in regular physical activity to improve overall health and fitness and to prevent negative health outcomes. The benefits of physical activity occur in generally healthy people of all ages, in people at risk of developing chronic diseases, and in people with chronic conditions or disabilities. This chapter describes an overview of research findings on physical activity and health. The accompanying box provides a summary of benefits.

Physical activity affects many health conditions, and the specific amounts and types of activity that benefit each condition vary. In developing public health guidelines, the challenge is to integrate scientific information across all health benefits and identify a critical range of physical activity that appears to have an effect across the health benefits. One consistent finding from research studies is that once the health benefits from physical activity begin to accumulate, additional amounts of activity provide additional benefits.

Some health benefits occur immediately after an episode of physical activity. Other benefits begin with as little as 60 minutes a week. Research shows that a total amount of at least 150 minutes a week of moderate-intensity aerobic activity, such as brisk walking, consistently reduces the risk of many chronic diseases and other adverse health outcomes.

The Health Benefits of Physical Activity—Major Research Findings

- ▶ Regular moderate-to-vigorous physicalactivity reduces the risk of many adverse health outcomes.

- ▶ Some physical activity is better than none.

- ▶ For most health outcomes, additionalbenefits occur as the amount of physicalactivity increases through higher intensity, greater frequency, and/or longer duration.

- ▶ Substantial health benefits for adults occur with 150 to 300 minutes a week of moderate-intensity physical activity, such as brisk walking. Additional benefits occur with more physical activity.

- ▶ Both aerobic and muscle-strengthening physical activity are beneficial.

- ▶ Health benefits occur for children and adolescents, young and middle-aged adults, older adults, and those in every studied racial and ethnic group.

- ▶ The health benefits of physical activity occur for people with chronic conditions or disabilities.

- ▶ The benefits of physical activity generally outweigh the risk of adverse outcomes or injury.

Examining the Relationship Between Physical Activity and Health

In many studies covering a wide range of issues, researchers have focused on exercise as well as on the more broadly defined concept of physical activity.

Studies have examined the role of physical activity in many groups—men and women, children, adolescents, adults, older adults, people with chronic conditions and disabilities, and women during pregnancy and the postpartum period. These studies have focused on the role that physical activity plays in many health outcomes, including:

- ▸ All-cause mortality;

- ▸ Diseases such as coronary heart disease, stroke,cancer at multiple sites, type 2 diabetes, obesity,hypertension, and osteoporosis;

- ▸ Risk factors for disease, such as overweight orobesity, hypertension, and high blood cholesterol;

- ▸ Physical fitness, such as aerobic capacity and musclestrength and endurance;

- ▸ Functional capacity, or the ability to engage inactivities needed for daily living;

- ▸ Brain health and conditions that affect cognition, such as depression and anxiety, and Alzheimer's disease; and

- ▸ Falls or injuries from falls.

These studies have also prompted questions as to what type of physical activity and how much is needed for various health benefits. To answer this question, investigators have studied three main kinds of physical activity—aerobic, muscle strengthening, and bone strengthening. Investigators have also studied balance and flexibility activities.

Aerobic Activity

In this kind of physical activity (also called an endurance activity or cardio activity), the body's large muscles move in a rhythmic manner for a sustained period of time. Brisk walking, running, bicycling, jumping rope, and swimming are all examples. Aerobic activity causes a person's heart to beat faster, and they will breathe harder than normal.

Aerobic physical activity has three components:

▶ Intensity, or how hard a person works to do the activity. The intensities most often studied are moderate (equivalent in effort to brisk walking) and vigorous (equivalent in effort to running or jogging);

▶ Frequency, or how often a person does aerobic activity; and

▶ Duration, or how long a person does an activity in any one session.

Although these components make up an aerobic physical activity profile, research has shown that the total amount of

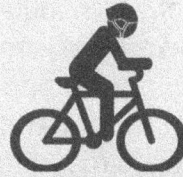

Physical Activity, Exercise, and Health

Physical activity refers to any bodily movement produced by the contraction of skeletal muscle that increases energy expenditure above a basal level. In the Guidelines, physical activity generally refers to the subset of physical activity that enhances health. Exercise is a form of physical activity that is planned, structured, repetitive, and performed with the goal of improving health or fitness. Although all exercise is physical activity, not all physical activity is exercise.

Health is a human condition with physical, social, and psychological dimensions, each characterized on a continuum with positive and negative poles. Positive health is associated with a capacity to enjoy life and to withstand challenges; it is not merely the absence of disease. Negative health is associated with illness, and in the extreme, with premature death.

physical activity (minutes of moderate-intensity physical activity in a week, for example) is more important for achieving health benefits than is any one component (frequency, intensity, or duration). All time spent in moderate- or vigorous-intensity physical activity counts toward meeting the key guidelines.

Muscle-Strengthening Activity

This kind of activity, which includes resistance training and weight lifting, causes the body's muscles to work or hold against an applied force or weight. These activities often involve lifting relatively heavy objects, such as weights, multiple times to strengthen various muscle groups. Muscle-strengthening activity can also be done by using elastic bands or body weight for resistance (climbing a tree or doing push-ups, for example).

Muscle-strengthening activity has three components:

- ▶ Intensity, or how much weight or force is used relative to how much a person is able to lift;
- ▶ Frequency, or how often a person does muscle-strengthening activity; and
- ▶ Sets and repetitions, or how many times a person does the muscle-strengthening activity, like liftinga weight or doing a push-up (comparable to duration for aerobic activity).

The effects of muscle-strengthening activity are limited to the muscles doing the work. It is important to work all the major muscle groups of the body—the legs, hips, back, abdomen, chest, shoulders, and arms.

Bone-Strengthening Activity

This kind of activity (sometimes called weight-bearing or weight-loading activity) produces a force on the bones of the body that promotes bone growth and strength. This force is commonly produced by impact with the ground. Examples of bone-strengthening activity include jumping jacks, running, brisk walking, and weight-lifting exercises. As these examples illustrate, bone-strengthening activities can also be aerobic and muscle strengthening.

Balance Activities

These kinds of activities can improve the ability to resist forces within or outside of the body that cause falls while a person is stationary or moving. Walking backward, standing on one leg, or using a wobble board are examples of balance activities. Strengthening muscles of the back, abdomen, and legs also improves balance.

Flexibility Activities

These kinds of activities enhance the ability of a joint to move through the full range of motion. Stretching exercises are effective in increasing flexibility, and thereby can allow people to more easily do activities that require greater flexibility.

Health Benefits Associated With Regular Physical Activity

Children and Adolescents

- ▶ Improved bone health (ages 3 through 17 years)

- ▶ Improved weight status (ages 3 through 17 years)

- ▶ Improved cardiorespiratory and muscular fitness (ages 6 through 17 years)

- ▶ Improved cardiometabolic health (ages 6 through 17 years)

- ▶ Improved cognition (ages 6 to 13 years)*

- ▶ Reduced risk of depression (ages 6 to 13 years)

Adults and Older Adults

- Lower risk of all-cause mortality

- Lower risk of cardiovascular disease mortality

- Lower risk of cardiovascular disease (including heart disease and stroke)

- Lower risk of hypertension

- Lower risk of type 2 diabetes

- Lower risk of adverse blood lipid profile

- Lower risk of cancers of the bladder, breast, colon, endometrium, esophagus, kidney, lung, and stomach

- Improved cognition*

- Reduced risk of dementia (including Alzheimer's disease)

- Improved quality of life

- Reduced anxiety

- Reduced risk of depression

- Improved sleep

- Slowed or reduced weight gain

- Weight loss, particularly when combined with reduced calorie intake

- Prevention of weight regain following initial weight loss

- Improved bone health

- Improved physical function

- Lower risk of falls (older adults)

- Lower risk of fall-related injuries (older adults)

Note: The Advisory Committee rated the evidence of health benefits of physical activity as strong, moderate, limited, or grade not assignable. Only outcomes with strong or moderate evidence of effect are included in this table.

The Role of Fitness in Health

Physical fitness is an important factor in the ability of people to perform routine daily activities and an important issue from a public health perspective. Physical fitness has been defined as "the ability to carry out daily tasks with vigor and alertness, without undue fatigue, and with ample energy to enjoy leisure-time pursuits and respond to emergencies."

Physical fitness has multiple components, including cardiorespiratory fitness (endurance or aerobic power), musculoskeletal fitness, flexibility, balance, and speed of movement.

Components of Physical Fitness

Cardiorespiratory Fitness	The ability to perform large-muscle, whole-body exercise at moderate-to-vigorous intensities for extended periods of time.
Musculoskeletal Fitness	The integrated function of muscle strength, muscle endurance, and muscle power to enable performance of work.
Flexibility	The range of motion available at a joint or group of joints.
Balance	The ability to maintain equilibrium while moving or while stationary.
Speed	The ability to move the body quickly.

A substantial body of research has examined the relationship between physical fitness—cardiorespiratory fitness and, in some cases, musculoskeletal fitness—and health outcomes. The findings show that greater physical fitness is associated with reduced all-cause mortality and cardiovascular disease mortality and reduced risk of developing a wide range of chronic diseases, such as type 2 diabetes and hypertension. To date, most studies were done in men, but new data indicate these relationships also exist in women.

Physical activity and physical fitness are related to each other, and both provide important health benefits. Increases in the amount and intensity of physical activity typically produce increases in physical fitness, particularly in those who are less physically active. The available evidence suggests that physical activity and physical fitness interact in their effects on a variety of health outcomes.

Some possible ways that fitness and health outcomes may relate to physical activity are:

- Physical activity leads to improvements in physical fitness, and physical fitness causes improvementsin health outcomes;

- Physical fitness may modify the amount of the effect that physical activity has on health outcomes; or

- Physical activity can lead to improved physical fitness as a health outcome.

The Beneficial Effects of Increasing Physical Activity: It Is About Overload, Progression, and Specificity

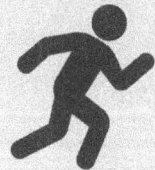

Overload is the physical stress placed on the body when physical activity is greater in amount or intensity than usual. The body's structures and functions respond and adapt to these stresses. For example, aerobic physical activity places a stress on the cardiorespiratory system and muscles, requiring the lungs to move more air and the heart to pump more blood and deliver it to the working muscles. This increase in demand increases the efficiency and capacity of the lungs, heart, circulatory system, and exercising muscles. In the same way, muscle-strengthening and bone-strengthening activities overload muscles and bones, making them stronger.

Progression is closely tied to overload. Once a person reaches a certain fitness level, he or she is able to progress to higher levels of physical activity by continued overload and adaptation. Small, progressive changes in overload help the body adapt to the additional stresses while minimizing the risk of injury.

Specificity means that the benefits of physical activity are specific to the body systems that are doing the work. For example, the physiologic benefits of walking are largely specific to the lower body and the cardiovascular system. Push-ups primarily benefit the muscles of the chest, shoulders, and upper arms.

The following sections provide more detail on what is known from research studies about the specific health benefits of physical activity.

All-Cause Mortality

Strong scientific evidence shows that physical activity delays death from all causes. This includes the leading causes of death, such as heart disease and some cancers, as well as other causes of death. This effect is remarkable in two ways:

▶ First, only a few lifestyle choices have as large an effect on mortality as physical activity. It has beenestimated that people who are physically active for approximately 150 minutes a week have a33 percent lower risk of all-cause mortality than those who are not physically active.

▶ Second, it is not necessary to do large amounts of activity or vigorous-intensity activity to reduce the riskof all-cause mortality. Benefits start to accumulate with any amount of moderate- or vigorous-intensityphysical activity.

Research clearly demonstrates the importance of avoiding inactivity. Even low amounts of moderate-to-vigorous intensity physical activity reduce the risk of all-cause mortality. A large benefit occurs when a person moves from being inactive to being insufficiently active. The relative risk of all-cause mortality continues to decline as people become even more physically active. Even at very high levels of physical activity (3 to 5 times the key guidelines), there is no evidence of increased risk.

Bone and Musculoskeletal Health

Bones, muscles, and joints support the body and help it move. Healthy bones, joints, and muscles are critical to the ability to do daily activities without physical limitations such as climbing stairs, working in the garden, or carrying a small child.

Progressive muscle-strengthening activities preserve or increase muscle mass, strength, and power. Greater amounts (through higher frequency, heavier weights, or more resistance) improve muscle function to a greater degree. Improvements occur in children and adolescents as well as in younger and older adults. Resistance exercises also improve muscular strength in persons with conditions such as stroke, multiple sclerosis, cerebral palsy, and spinal cord injury. Though aerobic activity does not increase muscle mass in the same way that muscle-strengthening activities do, it may also help slow the loss of muscle with aging.

Preserving bone, joint, and muscle health is essential with increasing age. Studies show that the frequent decline in bone density that happens during aging can be slowed with regular physical activity. These effects are seen in people who participate in aerobic, muscle-strengthening, and bone-strengthening physical activity programs of moderate or vigorous intensity. The range of total physical activity for these benefits varies widely. Important changes seem to begin at 90 minutes a week.

Building strong, healthy bones is also important for children and adolescents. Along with having a healthy diet that includes adequate calcium and vitamin D, physical activity is critical for bone development in youth. Children and adolescents ages 3 through 17 years who are physically active (such as by running, jumping, and doing other bone-strengthening activities) have higher bone mass, improved bone structure, and greater bone strength.

Regular physical activity also helps people with osteoarthritis or other rheumatic conditions affecting the joints. Participation in 150 minutes a week of moderate-intensity aerobic physical activity plus muscle-strengthening activity improves pain management, function, and quality of life. Up to 10,000 steps per day does not appear to worsen the progression of osteoarthritis. Very high levels of physical activity, however, may have extra risks. People who participate in very high levels of high-impact physical activity—such as elite or professional athletes—have a higher risk of hip and knee osteoarthritis, mostly due to the risk of injury involved in competing in some sports.

Functional Ability and Fall Prevention

Physical function, or functional ability, is the capacity of a person to perform tasks or behaviors that enable him or her to carry out everyday activities, such as climbing stairs, or to fulfill basic life roles, such as personal care, grocery shopping, or playing with grandchildren. Loss of functional ability is referred to as functional limitation. Middle-aged and older adults who are physically active have lower risk of functional limitations than do inactive adults. Physical activity can prevent or delay the onset of substantial functional or role limitations. Older adults who already have functional limitations also benefit from regular physical activity.

Hip fracture is a serious health condition that can have life-changing negative effects for many older people. Physically active people, especially women, appear to have a lower risk of hip fracture than do inactive people. Among older adults, physical activity reduces the risk of falling and injuries from falls. Research demonstrates that multicomponent physical activity programs are most successful at reducing falls and injuries. These programs commonly include muscle-strengthening activities and balance training and may also include gait and coordination training, physical function training, and moderate-intensity activities, such as walking. It is important to note that doing only low-intensity walking does not seem to reduce the risk of fall-related injuries.

The Benefits of Physical Activity for Brain Health

Outcome	Population	Benefit	Acute	Habitual
Cognition	Children ages 6 to 13 years	Improved cognition (performance on academic achievement tests, executive function, processing speed, memory).	●	●
	Adults	Reduced risk of dementia (including Alzheimer's disease)		●
	Adults older than age 50 years	Improved cognition (executive function, attention, memory, crystallized intelligence,* processing speed).		●
Quality of life	Adults	Improved quality of life.		●
Depressed mood and depression	Children ages 6 to 17 years and adults	Reduced risk of depression Reduced depressed mood.		●
Anxiety	Adults	Reduced short-term feelings of anxiety (state anxiety).	●	
	Adults	Reduced long-term feelings and signs of anxiety (trait anxiety) for people with and without anxiety disorders.		●
Sleep	Adults	Improved sleep outcomes (increased sleep efficiency, sleep quality, deep sleep, reduced daytime sleepiness, frequency of use of medication to aid sleep).		●
	Adults	Improved sleep outcomes that increase with duration of acute episode.	●	

Note: The Advisory Committee rated the evidence of health benefits of physical activity as strong, moderate, limited, or grade not assignable. Only outcomes with strong or moderate evidence of effect are included in this table.

*Crystallized intelligence is the ability to retrieve and use information that has been acquired over time. It is different from fluid intelligence,which is the ability to store and manipulate new information.

Cognition

Compared to inactive people, people who do greater amounts of moderate- or vigorous-intensity physical activity may experience improvements in cognition, including performance on academic achievement tests, and performance on neuropsychological tests, such as those involving mental processing speed, memory, and executive function. Physical activity also lowers the risk of developing cognitive impairment, such as dementia, including Alzheimer's disease. These improvements from physical activity are present for people who have normal as well as impaired cognitive health, including conditions such as attention deficit hyperactivity disorder (ADHD), schizophrenia, multiple sclerosis, Parkinson's disease, and stroke.

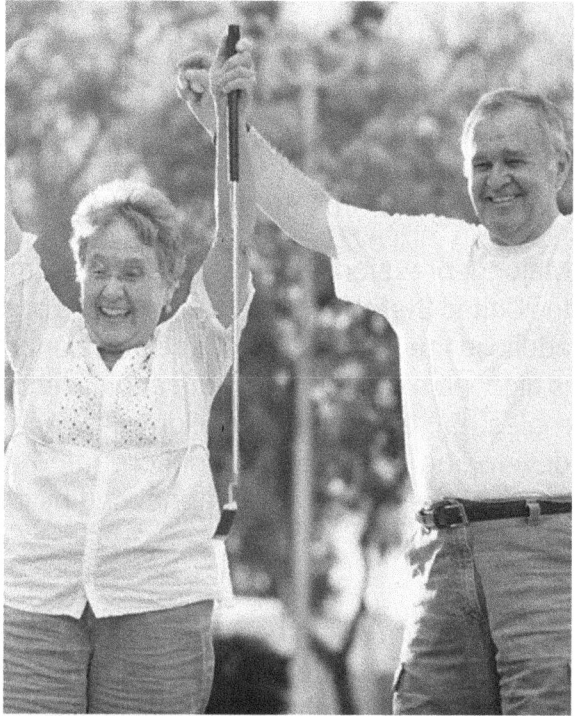

Healthy older adults, even in the absence of dementia, often show evidence of cognitive decline, especially on measures of processing speed, memory, and executive function. Physical activity may be an effective approach for improving cognitive function in older adults.

Quality of Life

Physically active adults and older adults are likely to report having a better quality of life. Being physically active also improves the sense of a better quality of life among people who have schizophrenia and related disorders.

Anxiety and Depression

Anxiety and anxiety disorders are the most prevalent mental disorders. Participating in moderate-to-vigorous physical activity over longer durations (weeks or months of regular physical activity) reduces symptoms of anxiety in adults and older adults.

Major depression is one of the most common mental disorders in the United States and is a leading cause of disability for middle-aged adults in the United States. The prevalence of depressive episodes is higher among females, both adolescents and adults, than among males. Engaging in regular physical activity reduces the risk of developing depression in children and adults and can improve many of the symptoms experienced by people with depression.

Sleep

In addition to feeling better, adults who are more physically active sleep better. Greater volumes of moderate-to-vigorous physical activity are associated with reduced sleep latency (taking less time to fall asleep), improved sleep efficiency (higher percentage of time in bed actually sleeping), improved sleep quality, and more deep sleep. Greater volumes of moderate-to-vigorous physical activity are also associated with significantly less daytime sleepiness, better sleep quality, and reduced frequency of use of sleep-aid medications. The improvements in sleep with regular physical activity are also reported by people with insomnia and obstructive sleep apnea.

The evidence that habitual moderate-to-vigorous physical activity reduces the risk of excessive weight gain, an important risk factor for obstructive sleep apnea, suggests that physical activity could have a favorable impact on the incidence of obstructive sleep apnea.

The number of hours before bedtime at which the activity is performed does not matter. Benefits are similar for physical activity performed more than 8 hours before bedtime, 3 to 8 hours before, and less than 3 hours before bedtime.

Cancer

Physically active adults have a significantly lower risk of developing several commonly occurring cancers, as well as lower risk of several other cancers. Research shows that adults who participate in greater amounts of physical activity have reduced risks of developing cancers of the:

- Bladder;
- Breast;
- Colon (proximal and distal);
- Endometrium;
- Esophagus (adenocarcinoma);
- Kidney;
- Lung; and
- Stomach (cardia and non-cardia adenocarcinoma).

These effects appear to apply to both men and women, regardless of weight status.

People With Chronic Health Conditions and Disabilities

Regular physical activity provides important health benefits for adults with chronic health conditions. Benefits exist for cancer survivors and people with osteoarthritis, hypertension, type 2 diabetes, dementia, multiple sclerosis, spinal cord injury, and other cognitive disorders.

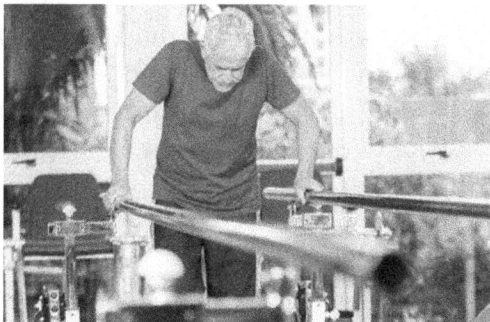

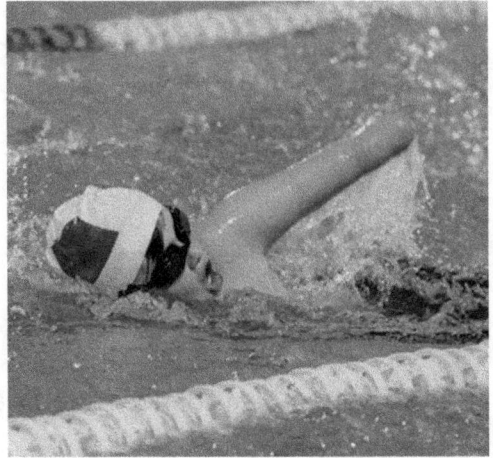

Adults who are physically active are healthier, feel better, and are less likely to develop many chronic diseases, such as cardiovascular disease, type 2 diabetes, and several types of cancer than are adults who are inactive. Regular moderate-to-vigorous physical activity also reduces feelings of anxiety and depression and improves sleep and quality of life. Even a single episode of physical activity provides temporary improvements in cognitive function and state anxiety. Adults who are more physically active are better able to perform everyday tasks without undue fatigue. Increased amounts of moderate-to-vigorous physical activity are associated with improved cardiorespiratory and muscular fitness, including a healthier body weight and body composition. Adults who are more physically active can more easily carry out daily tasks like climbing stairs, carrying heavy packages, and performing household chores. These benefits are true for men and women of all ages, races, and ethnicities.

Adults gain most of these health benefits when they do the equivalent of 150 to 300 minutes (2 hours and 30 minutes to 5 hours) of moderate-intensity aerobic physical activity each week. Adults gain additional and more extensive health benefits with even more physical activity. Muscle-strengthening activities also provide health benefits and are an important part of an adult's overall physical activity plan. This chapter provides guidance for men and women ages 18 through 64 years.

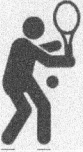

Key Guidelines for Adults

Adults should move more and sit less throughout the day. Some physical activity is better than none. Adults who sit less and do any amount of moderate-to-vigorous physical activity gain some health benefits.

For substantial health benefits, adults should do at least 150 minutes (2 hours and 30 minutes) to 300 minutes (5 hours) a week of moderate-intensity, or 75 minutes (1 hour and 15 minutes) to 150 minutes (2 hours and 30 minutes) a week of vigorous-intensity aerobic physical activity, or an equivalent combination of moderate- and vigorous-intensity aerobic activity. Preferably, aerobic activity should be spread throughout the week.

Additional health benefits are gained by engaging in physical activity beyond the equivalent of 300 minutes (5 hours) of moderate-intensity physical activity a week.

Adults should also do muscle-strengthening activities of moderate or greater intensity and that involve all major muscle groups on 2 or more days a week, as these activities provide additional health benefits.

How Many Days a Week and for How Long?

Aerobic physical activity preferably should be spread throughout the week. Research studies consistently show that activity performed on at least 3 days a week produces health benefits. Spreading physical activity across at least 3 days a week may also help reduce the risk of injury and prevent excessive fatigue.

All amounts of aerobic activity count toward meeting the key guidelines if they are performed at moderate or vigorous intensity. Episodes of physical activity can be divided throughout the day or week, depending on personal preference.

How Intense?

The key guidelines for adults focus on two levels of intensity— moderate and vigorous. To meet the key guidelines, adults can do either moderate-intensity or vigorous-intensity aerobic activities, or a combination of both. It takes less time to get the same benefit from vigorous-intensity activities than from moderate-intensity activities. A general rule of thumb is that 2 minutes of moderate-intensity activity counts the same as 1 minute of vigorous-intensity activity. For example, 30 minutes of moderate-intensity activity is roughly the same as 15 minutes of vigorous-intensity activity.

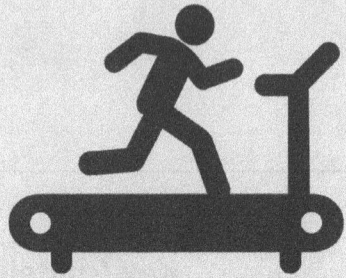

Offsetting the Risks of Too Much Sitting

People who sit a lot have an increased risk of all-cause and cardiovascular disease mortality, as well as an increased risk of developing cardiovascular disease, type 2 diabetes, and colon, endometrial, and lung cancers. The mortality risk related to sitting is not observed among people who do 60 to 75 minutes of moderate-intensity physical activity a day, but this amount of activity is far more than most people obtain. Therefore, both reducing sitting time and increasing physical activity will provide benefits.

The intensity of aerobic activity can be tracked in two ways—absolute intensity and relative intensity.

Absolute intensity is the amount of energy expended during the activity, without considering a person's cardiorespiratory fitness. The energy expenditure of light-intensity activity is 1.6 to 2.9 times the amount of energy expended when a person is at rest. Moderate-intensity activities expend 3.0 to 5.9 times the amount of energy expended at rest. The energy expenditure of vigorous-intensity activities is 6.0 or more times the energy expended at rest.

Relative intensity is the level of effort required to do an activity. Less fit people generally require a higher level of effort than more fit people to do the same activity. Relative intensity can be estimated using a scale of 0 to 10, where sitting is 0 and the highest level of effort possible is 10. Moderate-intensity activity is a 5 or 6. Vigorous-intensity activity begins at a level of 7 or 8.

Table 4-1 lists some examples of activities classified as moderate-intensity or vigorous-intensity based on absolute intensity. Either absolute or relative intensity can be used to monitor progress in meeting the key guidelines.

Table 4-1. Examples of Different Aerobic Physical Activities and Intensities, Based on Absolute Intensity

Moderate-Intensity Activities

- ▶ Walking briskly (2.5 miles per hour or faster)
- ▶ Recreational swimming
- ▶ Bicycling slower than 10 miles per hour on level terrain
- ▶ Tennis (doubles)
- ▶ Active forms of yoga (for example, Vinyasa or power yoga)
- ▶ Ballroom or line dancing
- ▶ General yard work and home repair work
- ▶ Exercise classes like water aerobics

Vigorous-Intensity Activities

▸ Jogging or running

▸ Swimming laps

▸ Tennis (singles)

▸ Vigorous dancing

▸ Bicycling faster than 10 miles per hour

▸ Jumping rope

▸ Heavy yard work (digging or shoveling, with heart rate increases)

▸ Hiking uphill or with a heavy backpack

▸ High-intensity interval training (HIIT)

▸ Exercise classes like vigorous step aerobics or kickboxing

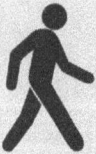

Spotlight on Aerobic Activities: A Tried and True Favorite and Two Increasingly Popular Options

Walking

Walking is an easy physical activity to begin and maintain as part of a physically active lifestyle. It does not require special skills, facilities, or expensive equipment. Many studies show that walking has health benefits and a low risk of injury. It can be done year round and in many settings.

Yoga and Tai Chi

Many different forms of yoga exist, and they range in intensity level from more meditative Hatha yoga to power yoga. For this reason, yoga may include time that would be characterized as light-intensity physical activity or as moderate-intensity physical activity. Yoga may also be considered both aerobic and muscle strengthening, depending on the type and the postures practiced.

Tai chi is typically classified as a light-intensity physical activity but may be considered relatively moderate intensity for some adults. It includes balance activities, and some forms may be considered muscle strengthening.

High-Intensity Interval Training

High-intensity interval training (HIIT) is a form of interval training that consists of alternating short periods of maximal-effort exercise with less intense recovery periods. There are no universally accepted lengths for the maximal-effort period, the recovery period, or the ratio of the two; no universally accepted number of cycles per session or the entire duration of the session; and no precise relative intensity at which the maximal-effort component should be performed.

When using relative intensity, people pay attention to how physical activity affects their heart rate and breathing. As a rule of thumb, a person doing moderate-intensity aerobic activity can talk, but not sing, during the activity. A person doing vigorous-intensity activity cannot say more than a few words without pausing for a breath.

Older or less fit adults may find that activities in Table 4-1 labeled as moderate intensity are experienced as vigorous intensity. These adults will gain health benefits from starting with activities that would be considered light intensity and, as they are able, to gradually build up to moderate- or vigorous-intensity activities. In contrast, younger or more fit adults may experience activities labeled as moderate intensity easy enough that they can sing while doing them. These adults may need to do more vigorous-intensity activities to gain certain health benefits.

> ## Talk Test
>
> As a rule of thumb, a person doing moderate-intensity aerobic activity can talk, but not sing, during the activity. A person doing vigorous-intensity activity cannot say more than a few words without pausing for a breath.

Muscle-Strengthening Activity

Muscle-strengthening activities provide additional benefits not found with aerobic activity. The benefits of muscle-strengthening activity include increased bone strength and muscular fitness. Muscle-strengthening activities can also help maintain muscle mass during weight loss.

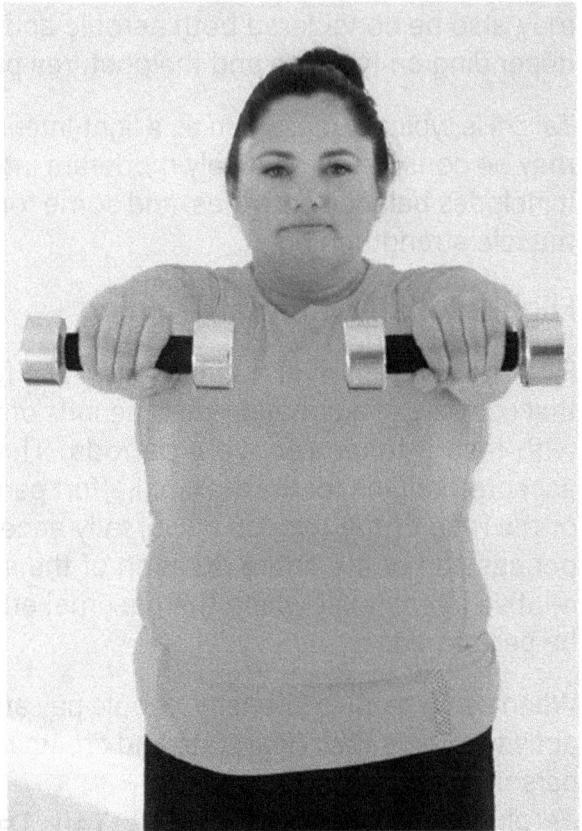

Muscle-strengthening activities make muscles do more work than they are accustomed to doing. That is, they overload the muscles. Examples of muscle-strengthening activities include lifting weights, working with resistance bands, doing calisthenics that use body weight for resistance (such as push-ups, pull-ups, and planks), carrying heavy loads, and heavy gardening.

Muscle-strengthening activities count if they involve a moderate or greater level of intensity or effort and work the major muscle groups of the body—the legs, hips, back, chest, abdomen, shoulders, and arms. Muscle-strengthening activities for all the major muscle groups should be done at least 2 days a week. The improvement in, or maintenance of, muscle strength is specific to the muscles used during the activity, so a variety of activities is necessary to achieve balanced muscle strength.

No specific amount of time is recommended for muscle strengthening, but muscle-strengthening exercises should be performed to the point at which it would be difficult to do another repetition. When resistance training is used to enhance muscle strength, one set of 8 to 12 repetitions of each exercise is effective, although 2 or 3 sets may be more effective. Improvements in muscle strength and endurance are progressive over time. Increases in the amount of weight or the days a week of exercising will result in stronger muscles.

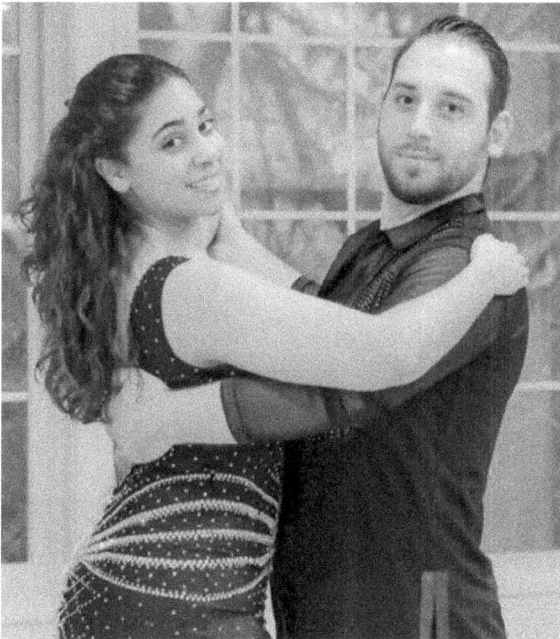

Flexibility Activities

Flexibility is an important part of physical fitness. Some types of physical activity, such as ballet or salsa dancing, require more flexibility than others. Flexibility activities enhance the ability of a joint to move through the full range of motion. Stretching exercises are effective in increasing flexibility, and thereby can allow people to more easily do activities that require greater flexibility. For these reasons, flexibility activities are an appropriate part of a physical activity program, even though their health benefits are unknown and it is unclear whether they reduce risk of injury. Time spent doing flexibility activities by themselves does not count toward meeting the aerobic or muscle-strengthening key guidelines.

Older adults should strongly consider walking as one good way to get aerobic activity. Walking has many health benefits, and it has a low risk of injury. It can be done year round and in many settings.

Table 5-1. Examples of Physical Activities for Older Adults

Aerobic Activities

- ▶ Walking or hiking
- ▶ Dancing
- ▶ Swimming
- ▶ Water aerobics
- ▶ Jogging or running
- ▶ Aerobic exercise classes
- ▶ Some forms of yoga
- ▶ Bicycle riding (stationary or outdoors)
- ▶ Some yard work, such as raking and pushinga lawn mower
- ▶ Sports like tennis or basketball
- ▶ Walking as part of golf

Muscle-Strengthening Activities

- ▶ Strengthening exercises using exercise bands,weight machines, or hand-held weights
- ▶ Body-weight exercises (push-ups, pull-ups,planks, squats, lunges)
- ▶ Digging, lifting, and carrying as part of gardening
- ▶ Carrying groceries
- ▶ Some yoga postures
- ▶ Some forms of tai chi

Note: The intensity of these activities can be either relatively moderate or relatively vigorous, depending upon an older adult's level of fitness.

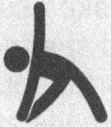

Yoga and Tai Chi

Yoga and tai chi are increasingly popular forms of physical activity.

Many different forms of yoga exist, and they range in intensity level from more meditative Hatha yoga to power yoga. For this reason, yoga may include time that can be characterized as light-intensity physical activity or as moderate-intensity physical activity. Yoga may also be considered both aerobic and muscle strengthening, depending on the type and the postures practiced.

Tai chi is typically classified as a light-intensity physical activity but may be relatively moderate intensity for older adults. Some forms of tai chi may be muscle strengthening. Research is currently exploring the effects that tai chi may have on balance and physical function in older adults.

Barb: An Active, 65-Year-Old Woman

Barb is recently retired and enjoys spending time being active with friends and family and at the local recreation center. Barbara does the equivalent of approximately 220 minutes of moderate-intensity aerobic activity each week, plus muscle-strengthening activities 2 days a week. Some of her active time is spent doing multicomponent physical activity.

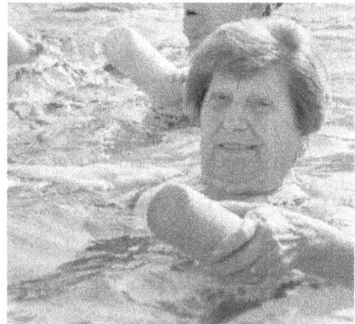

- ▶ Twice a week, Barb takes a 45-minute aqua aerobics class at the local recreation center with her husband. The class incorporatesaerobic and muscle-strengthening activities, and it helps her work on her balance.

- ▶ Many friends have begun to take dance classes at the local recreation center in the afternoons. Barb now joins them; she dances for 45 minutes and typically goes twice a week.

> ▸ In addition to her traditional activities, Barb makes sure to park farther away when running errands, and she tries to take the stairs whenever possible. These shorter bouts contribute an average of 40 minutes of relatively moderate-intensity activity to her total weekly amount.

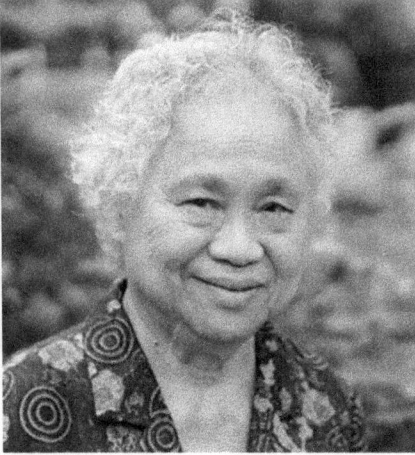

Rumi: A 79-Year-Old Woman in an Assisted-Living Community

Rumi struggles to stay active. She lives in an assisted-living community and no longer drives. She is worried about falling and heard from her doctor that staying active can improve her physical function and reduce her risk of falls and fall-related injuries.

Her goals and current activity pattern: Currently, Rumi walks 5 times a week in a loop around her assisted-living complex; this takes her about 10 minutes (50 minutes of moderate-intensity activity each week). Her goal is to increase the number of walks each week and also increase the length of some of her walks. In addition to her walks, Rumi goes with a friend to do bird watching with a group once a week at the local park. These outings usually involve at least 20 minutes of walking.

Starting out: Rumi slowly adds to her walks by taking a slightly longer route. After a few weeks, she is able to walk about 15 minutes 3 times a week. She continues to go to the bird-watching group.

Reaching her goal: Within a few months, Rumi is consistently walking the 10-minute loop around her assisted-living complex every day. She extends to a longer 15-minute loop at least 4 times a week. She continues to attend the bird-watching group, and she feels more comfortable walking on uneven terrain; she has extended these walks to about 40 minutes a week. Rumi has also started going to an exercise class for older adults twice a week. The leader teaches different exercises that focus on aerobic activity, muscle-strengthening activity, and balance training. Rumi is now meeting the key guideline of 150 minutes of moderate-intensity aerobic activity. This class has helped Rumi to meet the twice-weekly guideline for muscle-strengthening activities and adds multicomponent activities to her routine.

Getting and Staying Active: Real-Life Examples

These examples show how people with various health conditions can meet the key guidelines.

Jessica: A 28-Year-Old Woman Who Is Pregnant

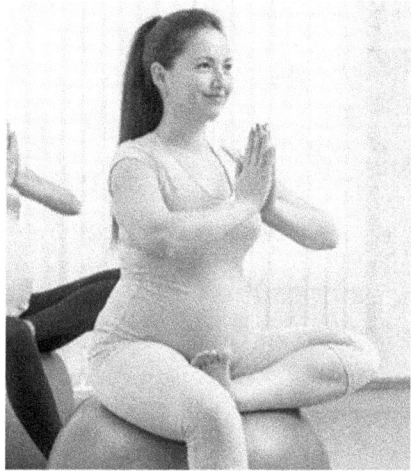

Jessica is 16 weeks pregnant, and her pregnancy is progressing normally. Before she became pregnant, Jessica did some light- and moderate-intensity physical activity, but she did not meet the key guidelines. Jessica's pregnancy motivates her to be more physically active. She discusses her plans with her doctor, who tells her it is safe for her to increase her activity level as long as she keeps him informed throughout her pregnancy. Jessica joins a prenatal yoga class at her local hospital, which meets once a week. She also starts walking during her lunch break for 30 minutes 3 days a week, for a total of 90 minutes of moderate-intensity activity. As she begins to gain strength and endurance, Jessica adds a 60-minute walk and 30 minutes of muscle-strengthening activities with resistance bands each weekend, modifying exercises to avoid lying on her back. With these additions, Jessica has reached 150 minutes of moderate-intensity physical activity a week and participates in 1 day of muscle strengthening. As Jessica's pregnancy progresses, she notices lower back pain that intensifies on longer walks, so she replaces her longer walk with swimming. She continues using resistance bands and attending her prenatal yoga class until her baby is born.

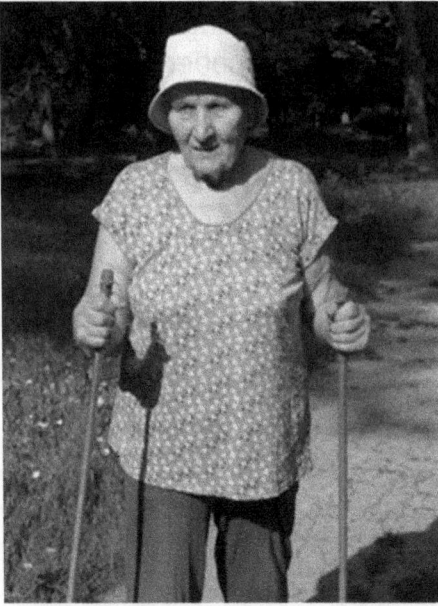

Ines: An 83-Year-Old Woman With Osteoarthritis

Ines has been active all her life, but osteoarthritis in her hip and knee have started to slow her down. Ines communicates regularly with her doctor, who agrees that staying active can help to reduce her level of pain, as well as improve her physical function and health-related quality of life. Because of her age and ability level, Ines typically judges the intensity of her activity based on her own level of exertion.

Ines does the equivalent of at least 160 minutes of moderate-intensity aerobic activity each week, plus muscle-strengthening activities 2 days a week.

▶ Three days a week, Ines follows along with a fitness video at home. The video includes 20 minutes ofmoderate-intensity movements, including stepping, marching, and walking in place.

▶ Two days a week, Ines participates in a 30-minute chair yoga class at the senior center nearby, whichincorporates muscle-strengthening, stretching, and balance exercises.

▶ On Saturday before the mall opens, Ines and her daughter walk for 40 minutes. The mall provides asafe, indoor place to walk with clear paths, even surfaces, and places to sit down if needed.

Chris: A 53-Year-Old Man With Multiple Sclerosis

His goals: Chris is a 53-year-old man with multiple sclerosis who sets a goal of doing 30 minutes of moderate-intensity aerobic activity on 4 days a week (a total of 120 minutes a week).

Starting out: Chris starts where he feels safe and comfortable, using a stationary bike at his gym. On the stationary bike, Chris does moderate-intensity physical activity for 20 minutes on 2 days each week. In order to track his progression, he takes note of his intensity level and tries to keep his level of effort at a 5 or 6 on a scale of 0 to 10.

Making good progress: Two months later, Chris is comfortably using a stationary bike at a moderate intensity for 30 minutes on 3 days a week. In addition to his time on the stationary bike, Chris has started to attend a water exercise class specifically for individuals with multiple sclerosis. The class focuses on multicomponent physical activity and meets one evening a week for 30 minutes.

Reaching his goal: Eventually, Chris surpasses his goal and works up to 160 minutes a week of moderate-intensity aerobic activity, including 30 minutes of stationary bicycling 4 times a week, a water fitness class for 30 minutes once a week, and a 10-minute brisk walk after work once a week.

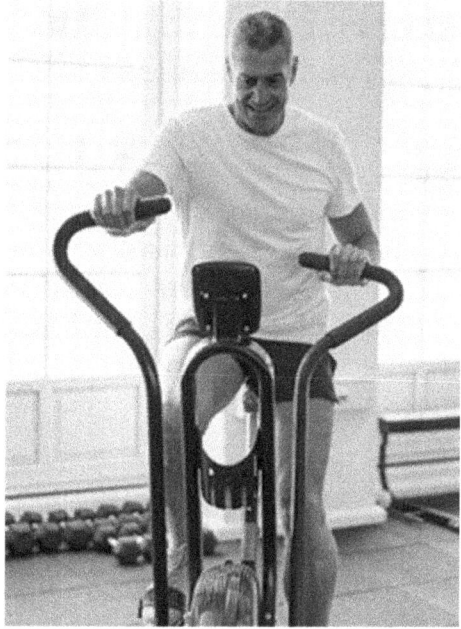

Raymond: A 42-Year-Old Man With Type 2 Diabetes

Raymond is a 42-year-old man with type 2 diabetes. Recently, at the recommendation of his physician, he started paying more attention to his activity levels. He received a step counter for his birthday, and he uses it to track his daily activity and stay motivated.

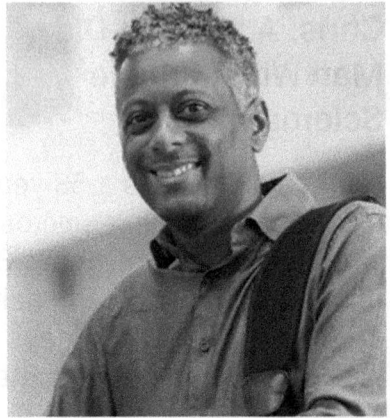

After a few months of increasing his physical activity, Raymond now does the equivalent of at least 150 minutes of moderate-intensity aerobic activity each week, plus muscle-strengthening activities 3 days a week.

- ▸ Raymond walks briskly to and from the bus stop each weekday(10 minutes each day).
- ▸ He walks with a coworker during lunch 3 times a week (25minutes each day).
- ▸ On the weekends, he and his wife ride their bikes to and from worship service (25 minutes).

Three nights a week, Raymond does body-weight exercises while watching TV after dinner. He does push-ups, lunges, planks, and squats.

Although physical activity has many health benefits, injuries and other adverse events do sometimes happen. The most common injuries affect the musculoskeletal system. Other adverse events can also occur during activity, such as overheating and dehydration. Rarely, people have heart attacks during activity.

The good news is that scientific evidence strongly shows that physical activity can be safe for almost everyone. Moreover, the health benefits of physical activity far outweigh the risks.

Still, people may hesitate to become physically active because of concern they will get hurt. For these people, there is even more good news: people can take steps that are proven to reduce their risk of injury and adverse events.

The key guidelines provide advice to help people do physical activity safely. Most advice applies to people of all ages. Specific guidance for particular age groups and people with certain conditions is also provided.

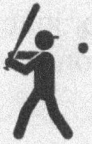

Key Guidelines for Safe Physical Activity

To do physical activity safely and reduce risk of injuries and other adverse events, people should:

✓ Understand the risks, yet be confident that physical activity can be safe for almost everyone.

✓ Choose types of physical activity that are appropriate for their current fitness level and health goals, because some activities are safer than others.

✓ Increase physical activity gradually over time to meet key guidelines or health goals. Inactive people should "start low and go slow" by starting with lower intensity activities and gradually increasing how often and how long activities are done.

✓ Protect themselves by using appropriate gear and sports equipment, choosing safe environments, following rules and policies, and making sensible choices about when, where, and how to be active.

✓ Be under the care of a health care provider if they have chronic conditions or symptoms. People with chronic conditions and symptoms can consult a health care professional or physical activity specialist about the types and amounts of activity appropriate for them.

Increase Physical Activity Gradually Over Time

Scientific studies indicate that the risk of injury to bones, muscles, and joints is directly related to the gap between a person's usual level of activity and a new level of activity. The size of this gap is called the amount of overload. Creating a small overload and waiting for the body to adapt and recover reduces the risk of injury. When amounts of physical activity need to be increased to meet the key guidelines or personal goals, physical activity should be increased gradually over time, no matter what the person's current level of physical activity. Here is general guidance for inactive people and those with low levels of physical activity on how to increase physical activity:

- ▶ Use relative intensity (intensity of the activity relative to a person's fitness) to guide the level of effort foraerobic or muscle-strengthening physical activity.

- ▶ Generally, start with relatively moderate-intensity activity. Avoid relatively vigorous-intensity activity,such as shoveling heavy snow or running. Adults with low fitness may need to start with light activity,or a mix of light- to moderate-intensity activity.

- ▶ First, increase the number of minutes per session (duration) and the number of days a week (frequency)of moderate-intensity activity. Later, if desired, increase the intensity.

- ▶ Pay attention to the relative size of the increase in physical activity each week, as this is relatedto injury risk. For example, a 20-minute increase each week is safer for a person who already does200 minutes a week of jogging (a 10% increase) than in a person who does 40 minutes a week(a 50% increase).

The available scientific evidence suggests that adding a small and comfortable amount of light- to moderate-intensity activity, such as walking 5 to 15 minutes per session, 2 to 3 times a week, to one's usual activities results in a low risk of musculoskeletal injury and no known risk of severe cardiac events. Because this range is rather wide, people should consider three factors when individualizing their rate of increase—age, level of fitness, and level of experience.

Age

The amount of time required to adapt to a new level of activity probably depends upon age. Youth and young adults probably can safely increase activity by small amounts every week or two. Older adults appear to require more time to adapt to a new level of activity, in the range of 2 to 4 weeks.

Level of Fitness

Less fit adults are at higher risk of injury when doing a given amount of activity, compared to more fit adults. Slower rates of increase over time may reduce injury risk. This guidance applies particularly to adults with overweight or obesity, as they are commonly less physically fit.

Taking Action

Improving the physical activity levels of Americans will not be a small task. Many partners are already involved, but more engagement is needed to increase the reach, breadth, and impact of these efforts. Realizing a shared vision of a more physically active and healthy America will require the dedication, ingenuity, skill, and commitment from many partners working across many different sectors. Being physically active is one of the best investments individuals and communities can make in their health and welfare. Now is the time to take action and help more Americans attain the numerous benefits of physical activity.

Getting and Staying Active: Real-Life Example

Jim: A 75-Year-Old Man Who Uses a Pedometer to Track His Increasing Activity

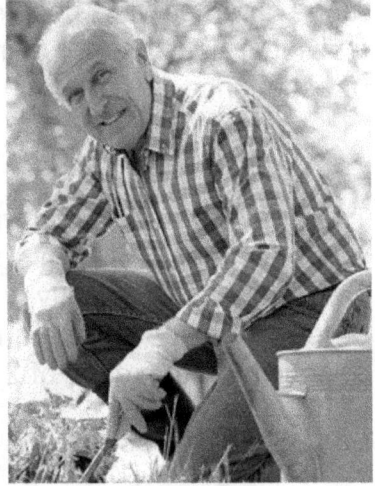

Establishing baseline: Jim does not yet meet the key guidelines, but he wants to increase his physical activity so he can continue to live independently in his own home. Jim spends 45 minutes each week taking care of his yard and garden. He also spends about 55 minutes cleaning the inside of his house, including vacuuming, cleaning bathrooms, and washing the floors. He is participating in 100 minutes of moderate-intensity physical activity each week.

Setting goals: Jim wants to add at least 60 additional minutes of moderate-intensity walking to each week. He purchases an inexpensive step counter to help set his physical activity goal and monitor his progress. Before starting to incorporate any extra walking, Jim wears his new step counter for one day and finds he gets 5,100 steps. He then wears his step counter on a 10-minute, moderate-intensity walk around his neighborhood and notes that this adds about 1,000 steps. Based on his initial activity, Jim sets a goal of adding 10 minutes of walking each day, which would add 6,000 extra steps a week with 60 minutes of moderate-intensity walking.

Reaching his goal: To reach his goal, Jim uses strategies like parking at the back of the parking lot when he goes shopping, walking to a nearby convenience store to pick up ingredients for dinner, or walking to a neighbor's house. Over time, he builds up to the equivalent of 160 minutes of moderate-intensity aerobic activity each week.

For more information and resources visit cdc.gov or hhs.gov.

www.ingramcontent.com/pod-product-compliance
Lightning Source LLC
Chambersburg PA
CBHW070119030426
42335CB00016B/2211